Current Opinion
COSMETIC DENTISTRY

Editor
J Golub-Evans
New York University College of Dentistry

Editorial board

Marcia Rita Adler (Brazil)
Carol Austin (USA)
Nathan S Birnbaum (USA)
Didier Cauchie (Belgium)
Gordon Christensen (USA)
William Dorfman (USA)
Ronald Feinman (USA)

George Freedman (Canada)
John A Kanca III (USA)
Sandesh Mayekar (India)
Michael B Miller (USA)
Derry F Rogers (Australia)
Rosa M Russian (Venezuela)
Kim Sperly (Denmark)

Published by Current Science
400 Market Street, Suite 700, Philadelphia, PA 19106

Copyright © 1995 by Current Science Ltd, Philadelphia.
All rights reserved. No part of this publication
may be reproduced, stored in a retrieval system,
or transmitted by any form or by any means without
the prior permission of the copyright holders.

ISSN: 1065–6278
ISBN: 1-85922-682-5

Film originated in italy by Sele & Color.
Printed in Hong Kong by Paramount Printing Co., Ltd.

Current Opinion in COSMETIC DENTISTRY

Craig Mabrito and Matthew Roberts	Porcelain onlays	1
Jonathan B. Levine	Esthetic diagnosis	9
Frank Celenza, Jr	Esthetic periodontics	18
Thomas S. Valo	Anterior esthetics and the visual arts: beauty, elements of composition, and their clinical application to dentistry	24
William M. Dorfman	Treating dental disharmony with mixed media	33
Kenneth L. Glick	Color management of cosmetic restorations	36
Jacqueline Dzierzak	Restoring the aging dentition	41
Debra Gray King	Methods and materials for porcelain veneers	45
William G. Dickerson and James H. Hastings	Indirect composite restorations	51
Frederick W. Costello	Porcelain veneer adhesion systems	57
T. Gary Alex	Advances in adhesive technology	69
Mark E. Ellicson	The high-tech dental office	75
Laurence R. Rifkin	A new esthetic impression system	80
Didier Cauchie	Repairing porcelain and ceramic materials	89
Harvey Passes, Morey Furman, David Rosenfeld, and Adrian Jurim	A case study of lasers in cosmetic dentistry	92
Richard N. Smith and Mary E. Naslund Smith	Marketing the cosmetic practice via television	100
David M. Schneider	Differing porcelain systems	107
	Index to subjects	114

Cover illustration: **Top**, A patient's smile before esthetic dental treatment. **Bottom**, The same patient after the placement of porcelain veneers. Treatment began with a three-step analysis of the patient's smile involving an esthetic evaluation form, computer imaging, and diagnostic wax-ups. This analysis provided the ground work for provisional veneers, which in turn served as a three-dimensional blueprint for the successful result. (*From* Levine, *Curr Opin Cosmetic Dent* 1995:9–17.)

CURRENT SCIENCE

Porcelain onlays

Craig Mabrito, DDS, and Matthew Roberts

Houston, Texas, and Idaho Falls, Idaho, USA

For years porcelain-fused-to-metal crowns have been the only restoration for posterior teeth in which strength and esthetics were important. Predictable results can now be achieved with a much more conservative approach—the bonded porcelain onlay. This article reviews the preparation designs as well as several types of materials currently available for the cosmetic onlay. An application using porcelain onlays to restore vertical dimension is explored. With this technique, moreover, the porcelain onlay is combined with porcelain veneer to achieve a functional and esthetic restoration.

Research continues to provide us with advances in adhesive dentistry. Recent literature contains numerous studies that present relevant information regarding the use of materials and techniques and their effect on adhesion and microleakage. Because this literature illustrates predictable bond strengths to enamel and dentin [1–14], many clinicians can confidently recommend the use of esthetic inlays and onlays.

The technique for these nonmetallic restorations has been thoroughly discussed by Jackson [15••]. This article should be reviewed as a basis for understanding the philosophy and technique of esthetic inlays. Following is a discussion of both the conventional and less conventional applications as well as the materials available for ceramic onlays.

Tooth conservation

One of the major advantages of a porcelain onlay restoration is its conservative approach to restoring weakened or missing enamel and dentin. Certainly most patients appreciate a restoration that removes no more of the tooth than is absolutely necessary to achieve the desired result. In general, patients and dentists alike want to keep as much natural tooth as possible while strengthening the remaining tooth structure. Too often, patients ask, "Why do you have to grind the tooth down to a nub in order to strengthen the tooth?" This makes little sense to them.

Patients also often think of crowns as terminal restorations for teeth because there is no other restorative option beyond the crown. Simonson (Personal communication) described the life of a tooth from the first small amalgam restoration through replacements with increasingly larger amalgam restorations, to an onlay, a crown, root canal therapy, and possibly extraction. Although this is often not the actual scenario, it has happened to enough patients to make many of them dread full-coverage crowns.

Once a crown has been placed, only another crown can replace it. Yet if an inlay or onlay fails, all of the options for treatment are still available. Patients seem to be much less concerned with the length of time a restoration will last than with having their dentist remove excessive amounts of natural tooth structure prior to that breakage.

Predictability

Personal experience since 1986 indicates that esthetic inlays and onlays have a longevity that is almost comparable to that of conventional ceramometal crowns. Despite the early design flaws, first-generation bonding agents, and the initial availability only of light-cured resin cements, the results achieved with these restorations have been extremely predictable (Fig. 1). If these results are extrapolated, we might have an indication of their potential life expectancy. Although 9 years of use is certainly not considered long-term in dentistry, the question may be asked, "How many of those same patients are driving the same cars they purchased at the time the restorations were placed?"

Tooth strengthening

Because the strength of a tooth restored with an inlay approaches that of the intact tooth, and the strength of a tooth restored with an onlay duplicates that of the intact tooth [16•], there are great indications for their use over that of a crown. Even if the esthetic restoration shows wear or breaks, the patient has had the use of the restoration during that time, and the technology will have advanced to the next level to provide newer, improved materials and techniques for the next restoration.

We have no idea how a possible replacement restoration will be designed or from what material it will be fabricated in the future. Advances in this area of dentistry have been significant and rapid. Patients often seem to understand this better than dentists and can accept restorations that do not last forever. The concept of potential impermanence can be referred to as *tooth banking*, in which a portion of tooth structure is held in reserve, available for future use.

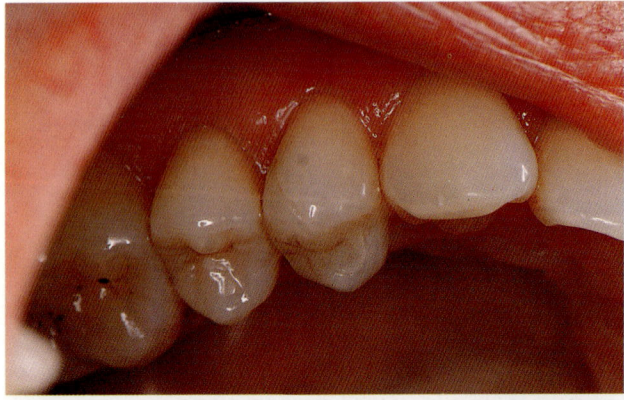

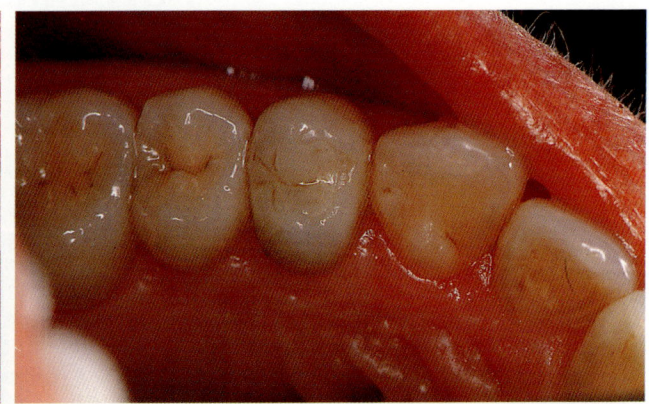

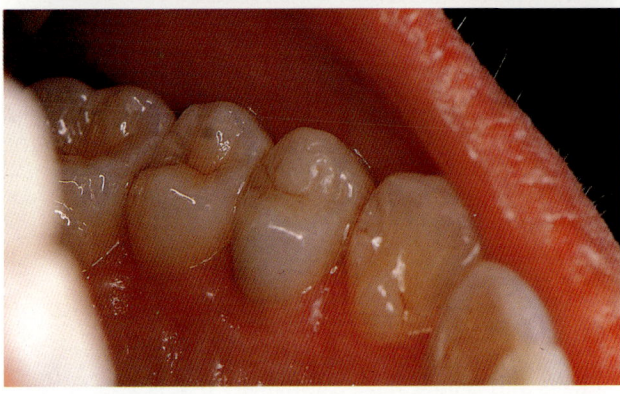

Fig. 1. Porcelain onlays bonded in August 1986 and photographed in October 1994. Although the marginal gap is visible after more than 8 years of use, it has probably stabilized.

Fit

Although porcelain inlays do not fit as accurately as gold [17••], they can be fabricated to provide an acceptable fit. The gingival margins of composite resin inlays have been shown to be between 24.5 µm and 28 µm [18•,19••,20,21•]. It is imperative that one use a qualified laboratory technician to achieve such results.

Because resin cements are used with bonded restorations [22••], the operator may tend to be less critical of the marginal adaptation. When a margin is less than ideal and the gap is filled with resin cement, the cement interface will wear, and the gap will open. After 1 year of use, these gaps between the tooth and the restoration will open owing to wear of the cement interface [23••]. The wider the marginal discrepancy, the greater the wear of cement, and the deeper the gap becomes. Consequently, as the marginal gap widens, it also deepens [24••]. Although this gap appears to be self-limiting, great care must be taken in the proper fabrication and cementation of these restorations.

Application

Restoring vertical dimension is one area of use for the esthetic onlay that has not been discussed at length. A decrease in vertical dimension owing to excessive abrasion or erosion can cause a collapsed facial form, chronic angular cheilosis, temporomandibular joint dysfunction, or myofascial pain [25•].

After proper diagnosis and verification of the corrected vertical dimension, esthetic onlays may be indicated for either virgin teeth or for those that have been previously treated with a restoration other than a crown. The advantages of esthetic onlays are the same as those of routine restorations of posterior dentition.

Why ceramic?

Because of their resistance to wear, high esthetic component, conservative preparation design (Fig. 2), and strength when bonded in place, ceramic onlays are the restoration of choice when vertical dimension is being restored and when a small restoration or no restoration exists in the teeth. Because ceramic full crowns are often involved in restoring vertical dimension, it is consistent to use like materials on opposing arches and throughout the entire mouth. Care should be taken to free balancing and working contacts in lateral excursions as well as to provide anterior guidance with posterior disocclusion when porcelain opposes natural dentition. This will prevent damage to the enamel (Fig. 3).

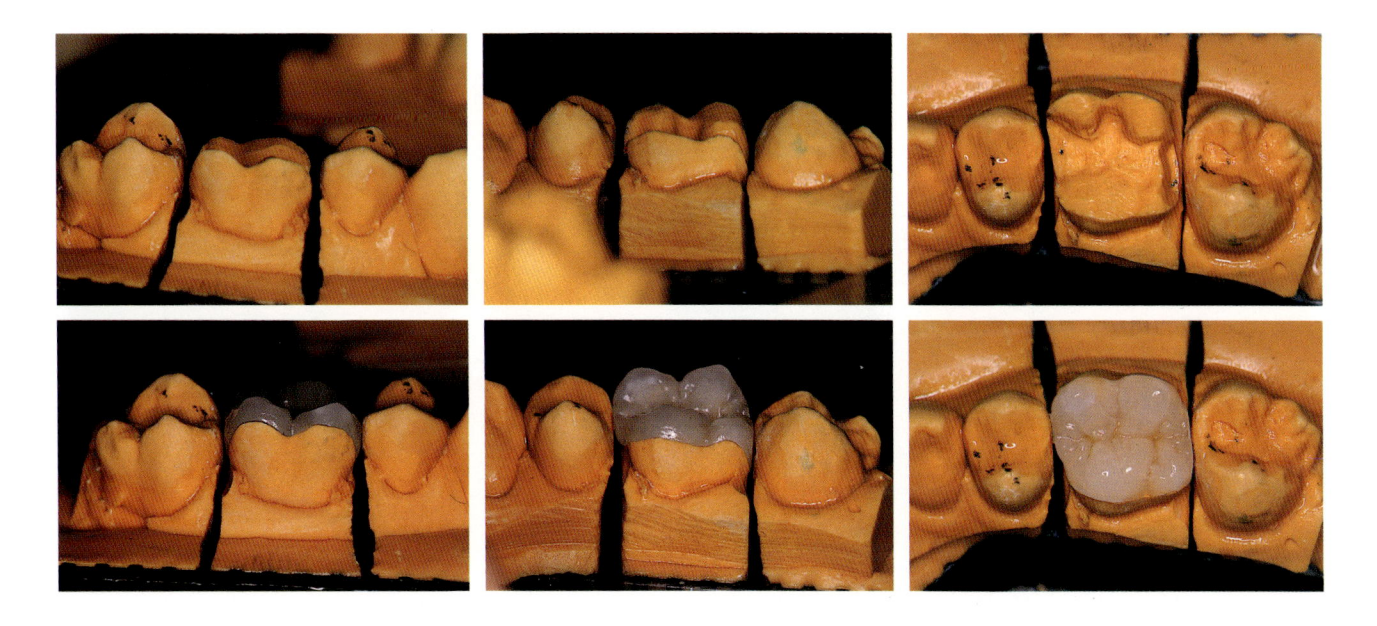

Fig. 2. Typical maxillary molar onlay preparations and restorations. Conventional resistance and retention forms used with cemented (*ie*, non-bonded) restorations are not necessary.

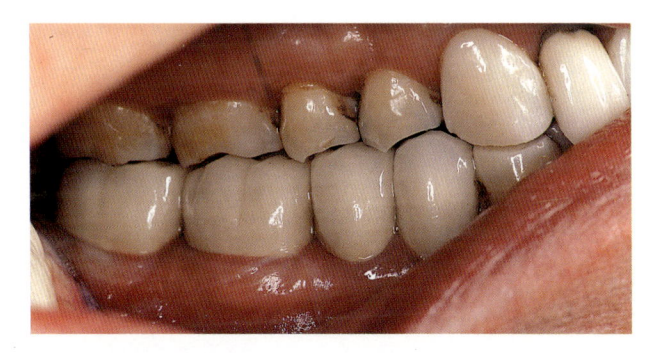

Fig. 3. Extreme abrasion of the upper teeth with poorly polished lower crowns and no posterior disocclusion in lateral excursions.

Preparation design

The preparations can be fabricated in the conventional form, *ie*, onlaying cusps where indicated for strength and appearance, or they can be combined with other preparations. This combination type of preparation is one in which the occlusal surface and the veneers are laid on the facial surface at the same time, which could be described as a reverse three-quarter crown.

When one prepares teeth for these types of restorations, careful thought must be given to the placement of the margins to allow proper tooth morphology. For mandibular teeth, both facial cusps and occlusal surfaces are in function and will need to be increased in vertical dimension to open the bite. This requires preparation of most, if not all, of the facial surface to allow proper tooth morphology. Placing the facial margin too far occlusally will result in a concavity at the margin area because of redirection of the buccal surface of the porcelain toward the now higher buccal cusp (Fig. 4*A*)

The lingual margin should be located at the height of contour or the most lingual aspect of the tooth. This is usually in the occlusal one third and leaves most of the lingual surface of the tooth unprepared.

In the maxillary arch, the lingual margin placement is the most common cause of problems (Fig. 5*A*). It needs to be placed far enough gingivally to allow proper contour of the lengthened lingual cusp. A preparation ending one third to one half of the way up the lingual surface works well for most teeth in normal occlusal relationships (Figs. 5*B* and *C*). Facial margins can be located in the occlusal one fourth of the tooth and still maintain good morphology. For esthetic reasons, most doctors choose to cover at least a portion, if not all, of the buccal surface (Figs. 5*D* and 6). Obviously, variations in occlusal relationship and orthodontic positioning can alter these guidelines (Fig. 4*B–D*).

Occlusal reduction will vary depending on the amount of the bite opening, but final restorations should be at least 1.5 mm thick in the areas of function, which is the very minimal thickness [26••]. No thickness appears to be too great; therefore 2 to 3 mm of porcelain is not considered excessive.

Both the onlay and the veneer have been made separately and in combination with one another. Cost is the main disadvantage of separating the two restorations, which requires two separate preparations, impressions, and laboratory procedures. For the small amount of additional reduction needed to achieve an acceptable path of draw, these two preparations can be combined to form this reverse three-quarter crown.

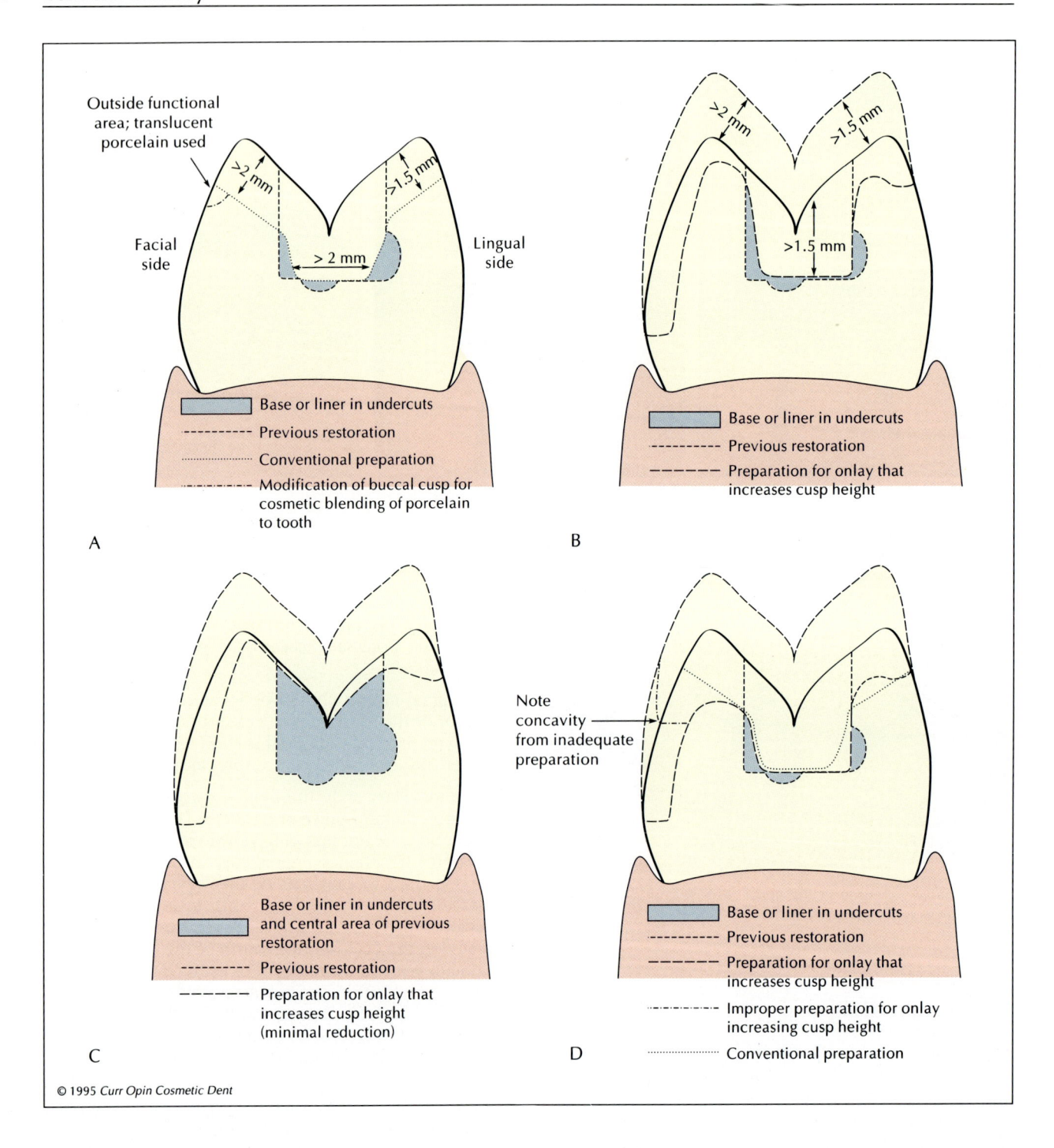

Fig. 4. Porcelain onlay preparation for a mandibular molar. **A**, Conventional preparation for the lower molar where the cosmetic blending of the buccal cusp is not a concern. Note modification for esthetics. **B**, Minimal preparation of tooth for an onlay that increases vertical dimension. **C**, Same as *B*, with modifications in the central groove area, blocking out all of the previous preparation. This preparation is easier for the laboratory to use. **D**, Preparation for an onlay that increases vertical dimension compared with conventional porcelain onlay preparations.

Ceramic selection

There are several options for selecting the material for esthetic onlays. Conventional feldspathic restorations have been used successfully, but we prefer one of the three high-strength porcelains, Optec HSP (Jeneric/Pentron, Wallingford, CT), Empress (Ivoclar-Williams, Amherst, NY), and Duceram LFC (Degussa, South Plainfield, NJ). Although this is an incomplete list, these are the materials with which we are most familiar.

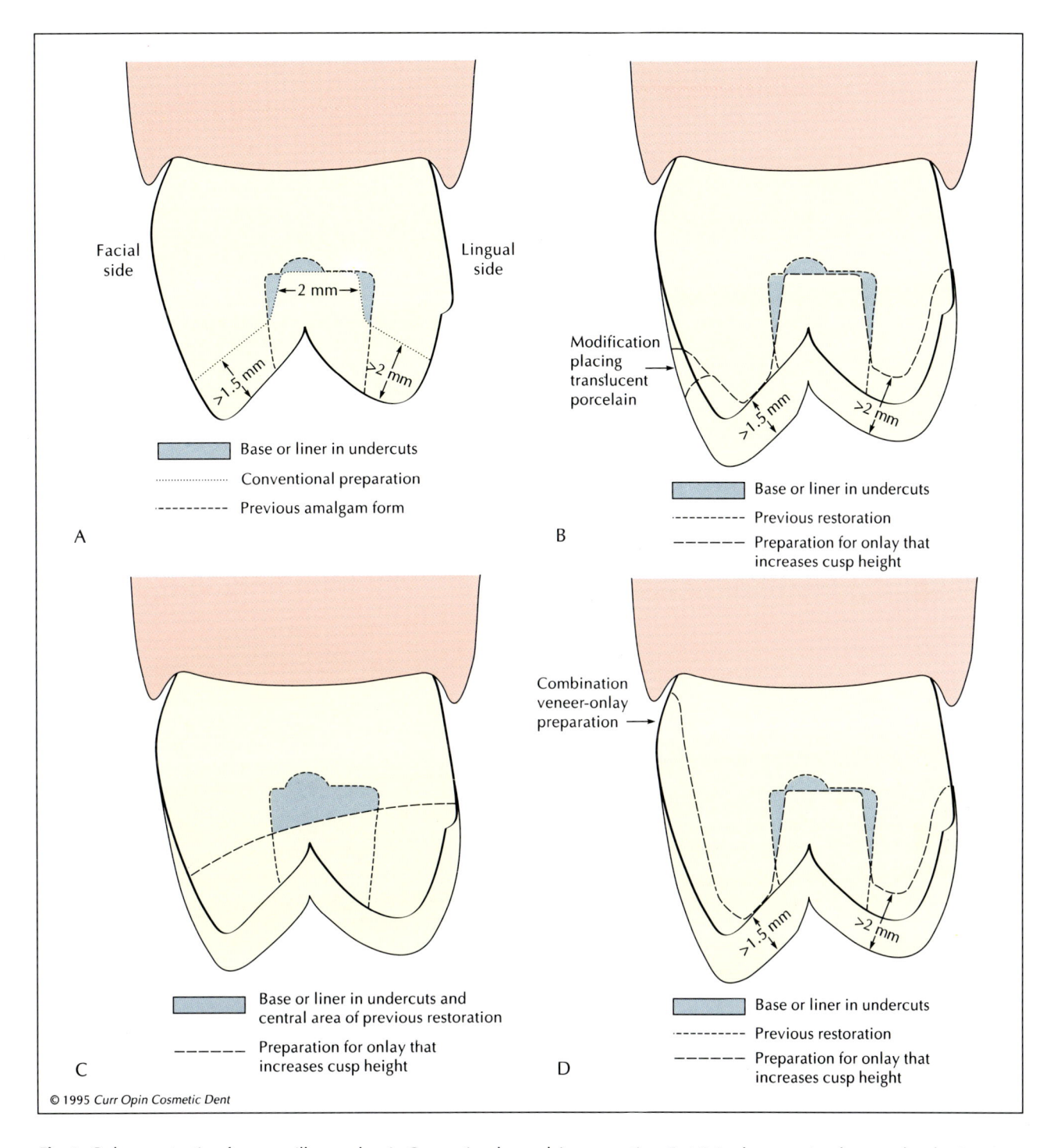

Fig. 5. Onlay preparation for a maxillary molar. **A,** Conventional porcelain preparation. **B,** Minimal preparation for an onlay that increases vertical dimension. Note modification for esthetics. **C,** Same as *B*, except that the preparation is more aggressive. **D,** Combination veneer-onlay preparation increasing cusp heights.

Optec HSP is one of the original Lucite-reinforced, high-strength porcelains. It requires a refractory die technique. It allows the use of a wet build technique to establish natural anatomy, the precise placement of internal stains, and the freedom to change the amount of translucency and color from one part of the restoration to another. Marginal accuracy is very good when the restoration is constructed properly. One disadvantage is that the use of a refractory die system makes achieving occlusal accuracy more difficult [27••]. Once the restoration is separated from the refractory material and placed back on the master model, it is difficult to stabilize, thus, there is less control in finalizing the occlusion. Moreover, once these restorations have been finished, the addition of porcelain to alter the occlusion is not recommended, and shades may not be modified.

6   Cosmetic dentistry

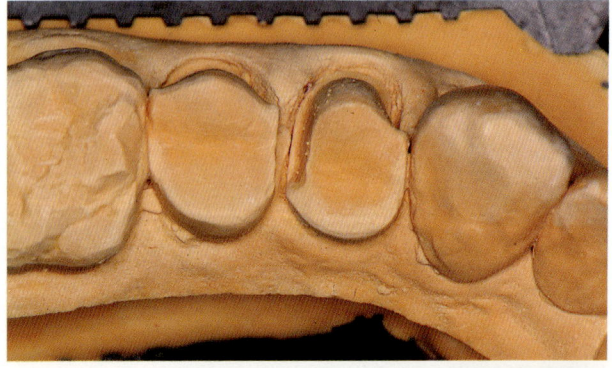

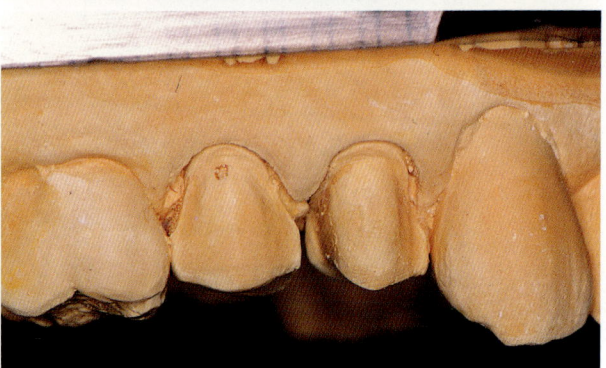

Fig. 6. Bicuspid preparations. Areas of decay or previous restorations can be included with the occlusal onlay and facial veneer preparation.

Empress has two separate techniques for use. Both use a waxed die and pressed porcelain technique that allows the use of conventional model and dye materials as well as more accurate articulation. There are four translucent levels of porcelain that are pressed to match any particular situation, which is were the two techniques vary.

The first technique uses the pressed porcelain as the actual restoration and surface colors and glazing to finalize the shading. The manufacturer claims that the color will not wear off because it is covered with a thick glaze. An advantage of this system is the ability to make shade changes without remaking the restoration, and because a wax-up is completed on the master cast, the occlusion can be fabricated with great accuracy [28••].

The second technique uses pressed porcelain as a core material similar to the metal substructure in a ceramomental restoration. Porcelain is baked around this core to form the occlusion, contours, and shading. Because this is all accomplished on the master model, the occlusion can be refined both before and after it has been tried in the mouth.

Although good marginal accuracy is obtainable with this system using either Empress system technique, it is not indicated for onlays unless there is significant reduction in the preparation. This system requires more room for the core and the porcelain overlay. Because the dentin shade of the margins' core material does not blend into the shade of the tooth, the preparations need to be subgingival where they are visible. This technique therefore lends itself more to the full-crown preparation.

Duceram LFC is a very low-fusing hydrothermal porcelain. It is highly esthetic, easy to polish, and higher in strength than conventional feldspathic porcelains. The manufacturer claims it is very kind to opposing dentition and that it increases in strength in the oral environment. Duceram LFC itself cannot be etched and bonded; it must therefore be applied over a layer of conventional, feldspathic porcelain that provides an etchable surface next to the tooth. Anatomy and color are built in wet (*ie*, before firing). The occlusion may be added after the restoration has been tried in the mouth. Color may also be modified at this time.

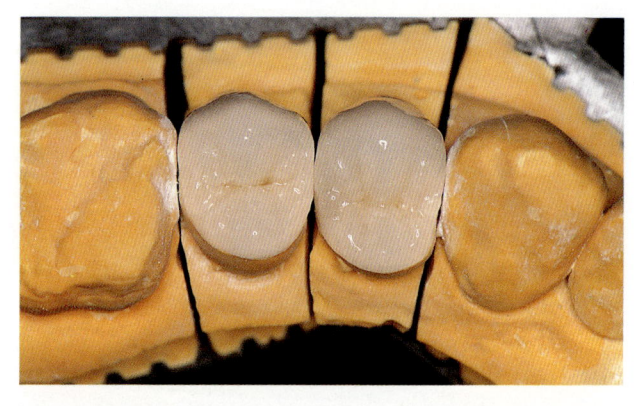

Fig. 7. Inspection of bicuspid restorations on working model prior to being bonded.

Other available materials deserve to be mentioned. The first is Spinell from Vident (Baldwin Park, CA), which is a new, translucent core material for the In-Ceram system (Vita Zahnfabrik, Bad Säckingen, FRG). It is not as strong as the original In-Ceram core material, but it is much stronger than the high-strength porcelains such as Empress and Optec. Spinell can be formed to an inlay or onlay shape with very accurate margins. Vita's Alpha porcelain is then baked over the core material to provide the color and contour of the restoration. The core material is nonetchable, and the manufacturer recommends Panavia 21 TC (J. Morita USA, Tustin, CA) as a cement. treating the core with Rocatec (ESPE-Premier, Norristown, PA) to provide a silica layer for silane and composite bonding is also being explored [29].

Composite resin

The other material that deserves comment is the indirect composite restoration. Although many have successfully used these restorations in onlay or full-coverage situations, we prefer porcelain. Composite is a superior restoration for inlays. Its advantage lies in ease of fabricating narrow, deep-inlay restorations, which owing to firing shrinkage, are difficult to make with porcelain. By definition, inlays have margins in the complex anatomic areas of the occlusal surface, and composite is easier both to finish here and to repolish than porcelain.

Occlusion

In general, the occlusion of bonded esthetic restorations is more difficult to fine-tune because of the die systems used and the potential inaccuracies in the bonding process (Fig. 7). In general, with bonded restorations the occlusion will be fine-tuned after the restorations are bonded in place. Consequently, we recommend restoring one arch at a time and finalizing the arch with the greatest number of esthetic onlays before completing the opposing dentition.

Sequencing

When crowns are opposed to porcelain onlays, the teeth may be more predictably restored with onlays prior to the completion of the full crowns. This may mean the upper arch is restored before the lower, or vice versa. Establishing the lower arch Spee's curve first may not always provide the most predictable results in the bonding of esthetic onlays. We suggest that the laboratory technician establish the opposing arch in wax or composite resin on the model. Then the restoration is made against this model, thus building in the proper alignment, Spee's curve and compensating curve.

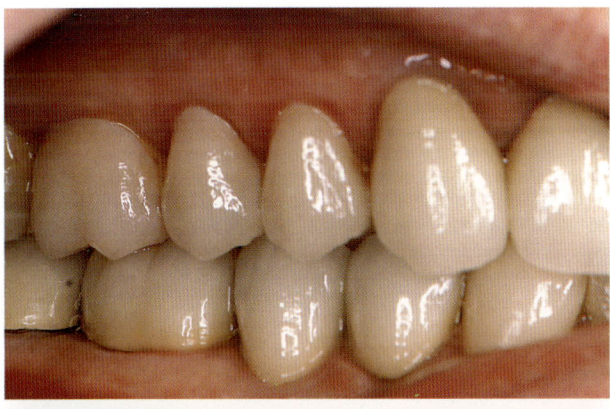

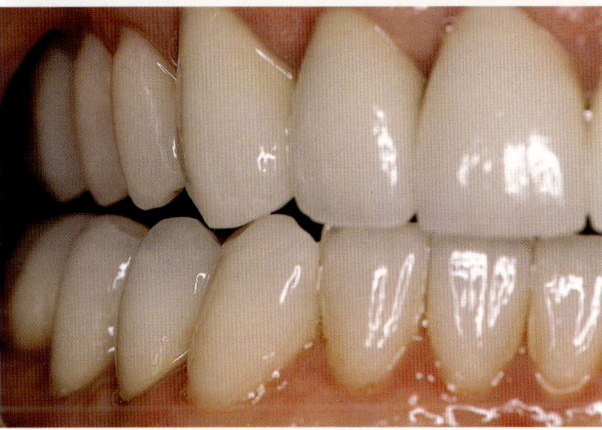

Fig. 8. Top, Completed bicuspid restorations with restored vertical dimension. Veneers were placed on teeth 2 to 5 and 22 to 27. Crowns were replaced on teeth 6 to 11 and 28 to 31. **Bottom,** Note anterior guidance in lateral excursion with disocclusion of posterior dentition.

Another alternative is to prepare all of the posterior teeth after establishing the proper vertical dimension. Both arches can then be built simultaneously. Again, at the chair, the arch with the greater number of onlays is bonded in place first. Then the arch with the greater number of crowns can be placed for a try-in, to make occlusal adjustments. If the occlusion needs additional alteration, a bite registration is made, and the laboratory can complete the occlusion.

Conclusions

Esthetic onlays provide another dimension to restorative dentistry. They strengthen teeth while conserving tooth structure. Not only are they strong, but they also replicate the beauty of the natural tooth. Because patients are more frequently requesting restorative dentistry that preserves their teeth and does not show like conventional metal restorations, we believe the use of porcelain inlays and onlays will continue to grow. With meticulous care, these restorations provide predictable results that can satisfy the desires of both the dentist and the patient (Fig. 8).

References and recommended reading

Papers of particular interest, published within the annual period of review, have been highlighted as:
- • Of special interest
- •• Of outstanding interest

1. Pashley EL, Tao L, Matthews WG, Pashley DH: **Bond strengths to superficial, intermediate and deep dentin in vivo with four bonding systems.** *Dent Mater* 1993, 9:19–22.

2. Davidson CL, Abdalla AI: **Effect of thermal and mechanical load cycling on the marginal integrity of class II resin composite restorations.** *Am J Dent* 1993, 6:39–42.

3. Perdigao J, Swift E Jr, Cloe BC: **Effects of etchants, surface moisture, and resin composite on dentin bond strengths.** *Am J Dent* 1993, 6:61–64.

4. Hadavi F, Hey JH, Ambrose ER, Louis PW, Shinkewski DJ: **The effect of dentin primer on the shear bond strength between composite rein and enamel.** *Oper Dent* 1993, 18:61–65.

5. Abdalla AI, Davidson CL: **Comparison of the marginal and axial wall integrity of in vivo and in vitro made adhesive class V restorations.** *J Oral Rehabil* 1993, 20:257–259.

6. Garcia-Godoy F: **Shear bond strength of a resin composite to enamel treated with an APF gel.** *Pediatr Dent* 1993, 15:272–274.

7. Ianzano JA, Gwinnett AJ: **Clinical evaluation of class V restorations using a total etch technique: 1-year results.** *Am J Dent* 1993, 6:207–210.

8. Ferrari M: **Directed shrinkage technique in class V composite restorations: in vivo microscopic evaluation and clinical procedure.** *Pract Periodontics Aesthet Dent* 1993, 5:29–36.

9. Van Meerbeek B, Mohrbacher H, Celis JP, Roos JR, Braem M, Lambrechts P, Vanherle G: **Chemical characterization of the resin-dentin interface by micro-Raman spectroscopy.** *J Dent Res* 1993, 72:1423–1428.

10. Ferrari M, Cagidiaco MC, Gesi A, Balleri P: **Preliminary report of an experimental design for in vivo testing of bonded restorations applied to a new enamel-dentinal bonding agent.** *J Prosthet Dent* 1993, 70:465–467.

11. Jordan RE, Suzuki M, Davidson, DF: **Clinical evaluation of a universal dentin bonding resin.** *J Am Dent Assoc* 1993, 124:71–76.

12. Kanca J: **Etchant composition and bond strength to dentin.** *Am J Dent* 1993, 6:287–290.

13. Abdalla AI, Davidson CL: **Shear bond strength and microleakage of new dentin bonding systems.** *Am J Dent* 1993, 6:295–298.

14. Barnes DM, Thompson VP, Blank LW, MacDonald NJ: **Microleakage of class V composite resin restorations: A comparison between in vivo and in vitro.** *Oper Dent* 1993, 18:237–245.

15. Jackson RD: **Esthetic inlays and onlays.** *Curr Opin Cosmetic Dent* 1994, 2:30–39.
••
This article provides the basis for understanding the materials, physical properties, case selection, preparation design, and complete fabrication technique pertaining to esthetic inlays and onlays.

16. Burke FJT, Wilson NHF, Watts DC: **The effect of cuspal coverage on the fracture resistance of teeth restored with indirect composite resin restorations.** *Quintessence Int* 1993, 24:875–880.
•
The authors tested fracture resistance of teeth restored with five indirect composite restorations. They found onlays were stronger than inlays with one group as strong as the intact control.

17. Molin M, Karlson S: **The fit of gold inlays and three ceramic inlay systems. A clinical and in vitro study.** *Acta Odontol Scand* 1993, 51:201–206.
••
This study compares three different ceramic inlay systems with that of gold. Gold was found to provide the best fit overall, and Cerec (Siemens Dental Corp., Bensheim, FRG) the worst.

18. Ferrari M, Mason PN: **Adaptability and microleakage of indirect resin inlays: an in vivo investigation.** *Quintessence Int* 1993, 24:861–865.
•
The authors evaluated the gingival margins of composite inlays for cement thickness and leakage. They found more leakage on dentin and cementum than on enamel.

19. Krejci I, Lutz F, Reimer M: **Marginal adaptation and fit of adhesive ceramic inlays.** *J Dent* 1993, 21:39–46.
••
The authors evaluated the marginal fit of several esthetic inlay systems after simulating five years of wear. The margins showed wear from chemical dissolution, toothbrush abrasion, thermal cycling, and occlusal function. The cervical margins had more wear than other areas.

20. Reid JS, Saunders WP, Baidas KM: **Marginal fit and microleakage of indirect inlay systems.** *Am J Dent* 1993, 6:81–84.

21. Milleding P: **Microleakage of indirect composite inlays: an in vitro comparison with the direct technique.** *Acta Odontol Scand* 1993, 50:295–301.
•
The author evaluated leakage in both direct and indirect composite inlays. He found bonded inlays had no leakage on enamel and the least leakage on cervical margins when compared with the other materials.

22. Hoglund C, Van Dijken J, Olofsson AL: **A clinical evaluation of adhesively luted ceramic inlays.** *Swed Dent J* 1992, 16:169–171.
••
The authors studied 118 Mirage (Chameleon Dental Products Kansas City, KS) inlay and onlay restorations cemented with either glass ionomer cement or a resin cement. They found a 2% failure rate with the resin cement.

23. O'Neal SJ, Miracle RL, Leinfelder KF: **Evaluating interfacial gaps for esthetic inlays.** *J Am Dent Assoc* 1993, 124:48–54.
••
The authors used six resin cements with four types of esthetic inlays to evaluate the occlusal marginal gaps. The cements showed wear mostly during the first 2 years. Dual Cement (Ivoclar North America, Amherst, NY), a microfill, had the least wear.

24. Kawai D, Isenberg BP, Leinfelder KF: **The effect of gap dimension on composite resin cement wear.** *Quintessence Int* 1993, 25:53–58.
••
This study evaluated the width and depth of marginal gaps using two hybrid and one microfill cement. Dual Cement (a microfill) had less wear than the hybrid cements. Moreover, the wider the gap, the deeper it became.

25. Dawson P: *Evaluation, Diagnosis and Treatment of Occlusal Problems.* St. Louis: CV Mosby; 1989.
•
This is one of the standard texts for understanding, diagnosing, and restoring teeth of patients with occlusion problems and symptoms of temporomandibular dysfunction.

26. Miller MB, Mabrito C, Castellanos I: **Porcelain and indirect resin inlays and onlays.** In *Reality, the Information Source for Esthetic Dentistry.* Houston: Reality Publishing Co.; 1993: 347–357.
••
This chapter on porcelain and indirect resin inlays and onlays provides an easy-to-follow and detailed technique. The ratings section is helpful when choosing materials for the procedure.

27. Molin M, Karlsson S: **A clinical evaluation of the Optec inlay system.** *Acta Odontol Scand* 1992 50:227–233.
••
The authors report the finding of 205 Optec inlays completed by 10 dentists in 57 patients. Among other findings, they rated 70% of the margins excellent.

28. Krejci I, Lutz F, Reimer M, Heinzmann JL: **Wear of ceramic inlays, their enamel antagonists, and luting cements.** *J Prosthet Dent* 1993, 60:425–430.
••
This study compared the wear of several ceramic inlay systems, including the wear on the porcelain, the opposing dentition, and the bonding cements. Polished Empress showed the least wear and caused the least opposing enamel wear. Dual Cement had the least wear of cements testing.

29. Kern M, Thompson VP: **Sandblasting, silicoating of glass infiltrated all ceramic: volume loss morphology changes in surface composition.** *J Prosthet Dent* 1994, 71:453–460.

Craig Mabrito, DDS, Park Plaza Professional Building, 1213 Hermann Drive, Suite 525, Houston, TX 77004, USA.

Matthew Roberts, CMR Dental Laboratory, 1400 East 17th Street, Idaho Falls, ID 83404, USA.

Esthetic diagnosis

Jonathan B. Levine, DMD

New York, New York, USA

> To ensure esthetic success, dental practitioners must respond to patient inquiries with a codiagnostic approach, allowing the clear identification of esthetic problems and the visualization of solutions. This structured approach involves a therapeutic mind set whereby a *common esthetic language* is established, and a communication triangle is formed between the patient, the dentist, and the technicians. The problem is clearly identified through the use of the esthetic evaluation form, diagnostic casts, and computer imaging. The solutions are visualized and treatment methods established through a diagnostic wax-up and computer imaging. This approach works by building a high-energy, high-trust relationship between the doctor and the patient, which serves to increase the probability of successful and consistent treatment and improves the dentist's general understanding of esthetic concepts.

It has been well-documented that the desire for improved esthetics and an enhanced smile motivates a person to seek dental treatment [1]. In today's dental marketplace, however, it is often confusing for patients to choose the right form of treatment. There are general dentists, cosmetic dentists, restorative dentists, and prosthodontists. What a myriad of choices, and what a competitive environment in which practitioners must operate! If we, as clinicians, are to be successful in the 90s, it is evident that esthetics must be a focal point of our practices.

When a patient inquires about esthetic improvement, the response requires a master diagnostician [2]. If consistent, successful results are desired, the principles central to avoiding remakes and esthetic failures must be understood. Interestingly, one of the major causes of failure is not technical problems but miscommunication between the patient and the dentist or technician. It is therefore necessary to incorporate the patient's perceptions of esthetics into the diagnosis. Patients must have the opportunity to converse with the diagnostician on proposed treatment. The outcome can then be visualized, and the patient can preview the proposal. This codiagnostic effort creates successful outcomes for everyone involved.

Most dentists diagnose esthetic problems using the classic steps of radiography and clinical examination and reach decisions based on their own subjective view of esthetics [3–5]. As Brisman [6] pointed out, patients and dentists all have varying opinions concerning smiles and esthetic looks. Romani *et al.* [7•] stated that professionals' opinions regarding evaluation of facial esthetics may not coincide with the perceptions and expectations of patients or lay persons. Therefore, the chance of inconsistent and unpredictable results is great.

This article offers a methodical three-step approach that allows the clear identification of esthetic problems and the visualization of solutions that will minimize failure. As Dawson [8] said 20 years ago, "If you know where you are and you know where you want to go, getting there is easy."

The structured approach

The structured approach involves three fundamental elements:

1. Developing a therapeutic mind set, *ie*, a systematic way of thinking about esthetic problems.

2. Understanding the fundamentals of esthetics, so that communication between patient and doctor is maximized. These fundamentals become the vocabulary for a *common esthetic language* between dentist, patient, and technicians. Without these fundamentals, everything is reduced to opinion.

3. With the knowledge of esthetics, and the esthetic language understood, the clinician goes through a methodical three step analysis of the patient's esthetic needs and desires.

The therapeutic mind set

A structured approach needs to be inculcated into our thought process whereby the esthetic problem is identified, and the solution is then visualized. Once these steps are taken, the appropriate technique can be chosen. In this way, technique-driven diagnosis is eliminated, *ie*, because solutions are visualized, we cannot simply resort to our favorite methodology but must decide on a course of action that intelligently achieves the visualized solution. After going through these methodical steps, the dentist can choose appropriate techniques for consistent results.

The common esthetic language

The common esthetic language uses the fundamentals of esthetics as its vocabulary. Dental esthetics, first described by Lombardi [9] in 1974, is defined by the way things are perceived visually. This visual perception at times is quite subjective, but if esthetic problems are to be handled in a predictable manner, "objective" thoughts must be established in order to have a starting point for an esthetic communication between the patient, the dentist, and the technician. The following discussion defines some of the important elements.

Visual perception can be divided into two categories: composition and proportion. Composition is the way color, contour, and texture relate to one another. Proportion is defined as balance, symmetry, parallel lines, curves, and how they work together. The esthetics of the face encompasses three views: the facial view, the dentofacial view, and the dental view. The following discussion serves only as a summary of these views.

The paramount element of the facial view is the midline, which acts as the centering vertical line. Organized around this midline and perpendicular to it are horizontal reference lines: the hair line, the ophriac line (eyebrows), the interpupillary line, the interalar line, and the commissural line. According to Golub [10], "The dental midline runs perpendicular to the interpupillary lines and serves to anchor the smile on the face." In addition, the general direction of the incisal plane of the maxillary teeth and the gingival margin outline must parallel the interpupillary line. This harmony must be reinforced by the incisal plane's following the lower lip during smiling. According to Chiche and Pinault [11**], strict parallelism between the elements is not required; it must be determined, however, whether they conflict with, or are not supportive of, the general horizontal perspective of the face. If this conflict occurs, it is critical for the dentist to observe the canting of the maxilla at the diagnostic phase, because this will affect the progression of treatment.

In a profile view, the nasolabial angle and Rickett's E-plane indicate where the lips are in relation to the rest of the face. Lip position (either prominent or receding) affects the shape and position of the upper anterior teeth and is consequently an important element to consider. In general, a prominent upper arch (*ie*, a convex profile) requires the reduction in size of the upper anterior teeth. A receded upper arch (*ie*, a concave profile) calls for more prominent positions of teeth. Spear (Paper presented at the American Academy of Esthetic Dentistry 16th Annual Meeting, Santa Barbara, 1991) called this relationship *facially generated treatment planning*.

The dentofacial view involves the teeth and the surrounding structures of the gingiva and the lips. Rufenacht [12] described this view as a coincidence of curves created by the contact points, incisal edges, and the lower lip. It is important to evaluate the amount of tooth exposure in smiling and at rest. According to Tjan and Miller [13], the average smile reveals 75% to 100% of the maxillary anterior tooth; the incisal curve of the teeth should be parallel to the lower lip, and the incisal curve of the maxillary teeth should be slightly missing or touching the lower premolars. Vig and Brundo [14] demonstrated that the mandibular incisor display in patients over 60 years of age should be approximately equal to the maxillary incisor display in patients under 30 years of age. On average, moreover, women exposed twice as much maxillary tooth as men (3.4 vs 1.91 mm).

Gingival symmetry at the midline is critical for the patient with a moderate to high smile line and needs careful evaluation [15]. Phonetics also need to be analyzed in this view, because a tremendous range exists between patients with varying occlusions. The "f" and "v" sounds help to determine the incisal third position, and the "s" serves as the guide for vertical dimension and the closest speaking space [16].

Viewed in the dentofacial perspective, the midline needs to coincide with the median lip of the philtrum [17] and should be parallel to the imaginary line dividing the face. The problems occur when the midline is turned off to one side. It appears that the vertical position, and not the precise mesiodistal position, is important. In summary, the perfect smile is aligned with the interpupillary line and centered on a perpendicular midline.

The dental view relates to the teeth and the gingiva and is defined by contour, texture, color, and proportion. Contour can be further broken down into its important elements of axial inclination, line angles (ie, contour ridges), heights of contour, incisal edge contour and position, and gingival contour [18]. Geometrically, anterior teeth are trigonal, with the height of contour (viewed incisoapically) distal to a line running vertically through the middle of the tooth. The mesial line angles of the central teeth mirror each other to create symmetry at the midline [19], and this is reinforced by an even gingival height. The axial inclinations of the anterior teeth are directed distally.

Proportion is defined by both tooth proportion and tooth-to-tooth proportion. Tooth-to-tooth proportion is guided by the law of the golden proportion: the ratio of the width of the central incisor to that of the lateral incisor to that of the cuspid, which has been defined as 1.6 to 1.0 to 0.6 [20]. Dominance of the central incisor is paramount in good dental esthetics, however, and the golden rule should be viewed with this point in mind. Tooth proportion is defined as the width-to-height ratio of the central incisor alone. This ratio should be between 75% to 80%. Anything less will give a long narrow tooth; anything more will give a short wide tooth [11••].

The three-step analysis

Once the common esthetic language is formulated, a structured, objective approach to the evaluation and diagnosis of anterior esthetics can be developed. This three-step analysis includes the esthetic evaluation forms, computer imaging, and a diagnostic wax-up.

To identify problems, a comprehensive diagnostic form is used (Fig. 1). The form begins by asking effective questions regarding what the patient would like to change about his or her smile. A careful analysis of three views is then performed. Facial symmetry, lip symmetry, smile line, horizontal and vertical tooth display, midline, and tooth contour are reviewed in a checklist style.

The next step involves the computer imager (Fig. 2). This task *must* be performed by the practitioner and not passed on to an assistant, hygienist, or associate. The procedure is a critical learning experience wherein the dentist brings his or her knowledge of esthetics to bear and, more important, involves the patient in the identification of the problems and the visualizing of solutions.

The patient is seated in front of the screen, and a professional-quality "before" picture is taken using the proper lighting, angulation, and camera distance. A key principle in this process lies in overcoming the patient's resistance to being told what to do and how to do it. The ideas people will support most are the ones they come up with themselves. The dentist must therefore ask effective questions [21], listen carefully, and respond to the patient's answers. The most effective questions are open-ended and encourage patients to express themselves. A closed-ended question only discourages patients from thinking and talking and elicits only limited information. For example, an effective question might be, "If you could change anything about your smile, what would it be?" A question that elicits a defensive yes or no—such as "Do you like your smile?"—would be ineffective. Effective questions establish a stronger relationship between doctor and patient; the patient feels empowered.

Effective listening is as important as asking the right questions [22,23]. A good rule of thumb is to listen 80% of the time and speak 20% of the time. This communication guides the doctor and patient to a high-energy, high-trust relationship in which patients are encouraged to identify their wants and needs.

The computer will produce two images: one that is unaltered and one that will show the proposed changes. Specific requests can now be made by the patient. The patient can ask a variety of questions, such as whether a gap can be closed, if teeth can be made lighter, or if the amount of gumline can be reduced. The effective questions will move from the broad to the specific, as solutions are visualized. As the dialogue proceeds, the dentist makes changes on the proposed-image side of the screen. Only a few minutes should be required for a proposed image to be completed and agreed upon.

A study cast is then taken, and a diagnostic wax-up is made to verify the proposed changes (Fig. 3). Some basic rules for the diagnostic wax-up are based on the fundamentals of esthetics:

1. Start with the central incisor and develop proper dominance (a width-to-height ratio of 80%). The prescription from the dentist must give information concerning the tooth length as determined by the esthetic evaluation form and the computer imager.

2. There must be symmetry at the midline, gingiva height, and contours of the central incisors. (Central line angles mirror each other.)

12 Cosmetic dentistry

Esthetic Evaluation

Patient _____   Examiner _____   Date _____

1. Effective Questions (E.Q.)

A. If there was anything you could change about your smile, what would it be?
_____
_____
_____
_____

B. Do you like the Media Image of "perfectly straight, white" looking teeth, or are you content with "healthy, clean, natural" looking teeth?
   ☐ Media Image   ☐ Natural Looking

C. History of esthetic change.
_____
_____
_____

D. Previous Records...
   Do you have previous photographs of your smile to aid in your Esthetic Treatment Planning?
   ☐ Yes   ☐ No

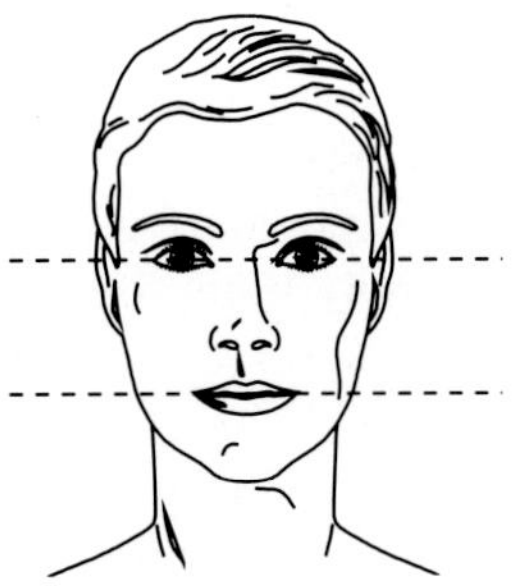

2. Facial Analysis

A. Full Smile
   1. Interpupillary Line to Occlusal Plane
      ☐ Parallel   ☐ Canted Right   ☐ Canted Left
   2. Midline Relationship of Teeth (Central Incisor) to Face (Philtrum)
      ☐ Symmetric   ☐ Right of Center ☐ Left of Center
   3. Relationship of Lips to Face (Lip Symmetry)
      ☐ Symmetric   ☐ Right of Center ☐ Left of Center

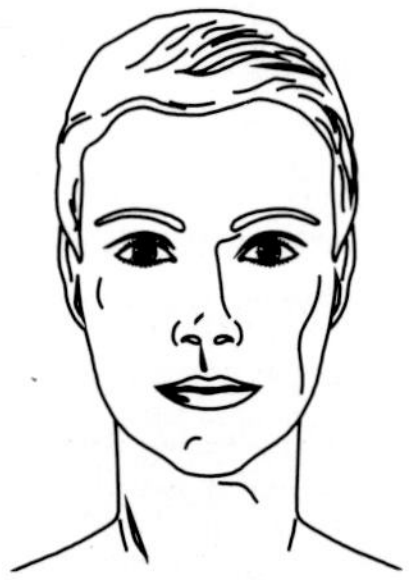

B. Lips at Rest
   1. Upper Lip
      ☐ Full   ☐ Average   ☐ Thin
   2. Lower Lip
      ☐ Full   ☐ Average   ☐ Thin
   3. Lips
      ☐ Prominent   ☐ Retruded
   4. Tooth Exposure at Rest
      Upper_____mm   Lower_____mm

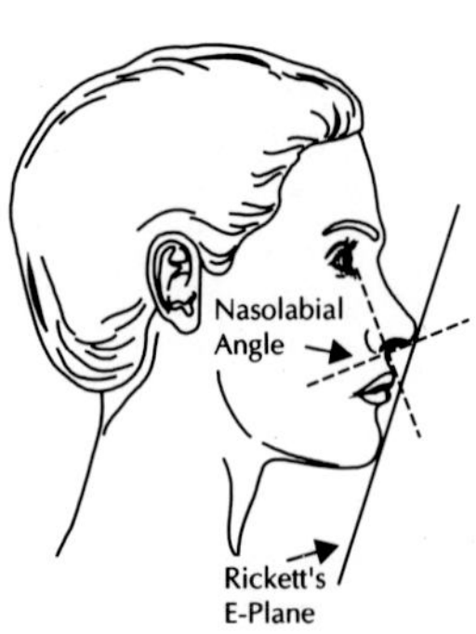

C. Profile
   1. Nasolabial Angle
      ☐ Normal approximately 90°   ☐ Prominent Maxilla <90°   ☐ Retruded Maxilla >90°
   2. Rickett's E-Plane
      Draw from Tip of Nose to Chin. Measure Upper Lip to E-Plane and Lower Lip to E-Plane.
      – Upper Lip 4 mm to E-Plane
      – Lower Lip 2 mm to E-Plane
      ☐ WNL   ☐ Convex   ☐ Concave

      If Maxilla is prominent, Nasolabial angle is <90°, or Profile is Convex...
      consider smaller, less dominant maxillary anterior restorations.

      If Maxilla is retruded, Nasolabial angle is >90°, or Profile is Concave...
      consider more dominant, labially placed maxillary anterior restorations.

Fig. 1. The esthetic evaluation form (*beginning*). The interviewing process begins with the asking of effective questions that encourage patients to identify their wants and needs. Three facial views are analyzed, and the prospective cosmetic work is related to the distinctive facial characteristics of the patient. WNL—within normal limits.

3. Dentofacial Analysis... Smile Type

    A. Upper Lip
        ☐ Average   ☐ High 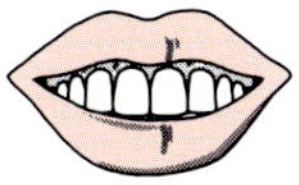   ☐ Low

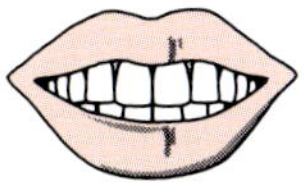

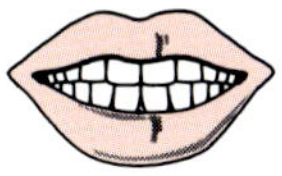

    B. Incisal Edge to Lower Lip
        ☐ Convex Curve   ☐ Straight 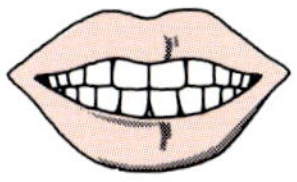   ☐ Reverse

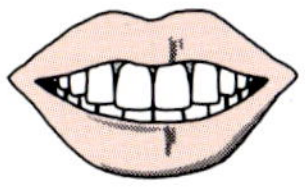

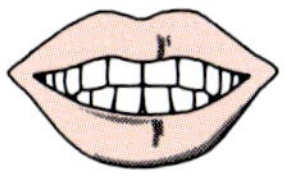

    C. Tooth–Lower Lip Position
        ☐ Touching   ☐ Not touching 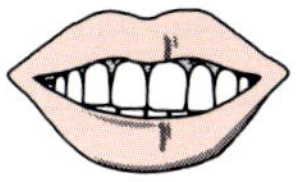   ☐ Slightly Covered

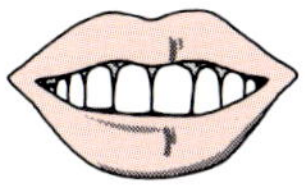

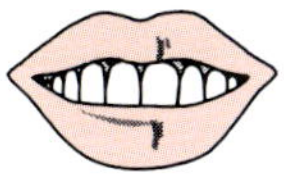

    D. Full Smile... How many teeth are exposed?
        ☐ 6   ☐ 8 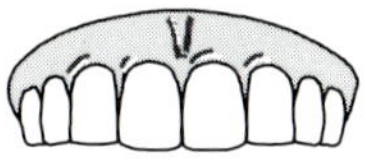   ☐ 10 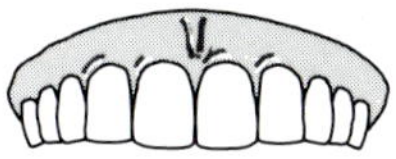   ☐ 16

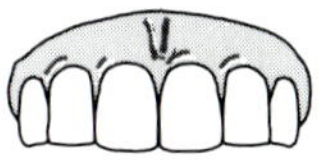

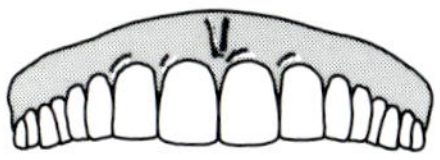

    E. Midline... Relationship of Central Incisors to Philtrum
        ☐ Center   ☐ Right of Center 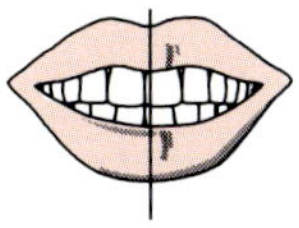   ☐ Left of Center

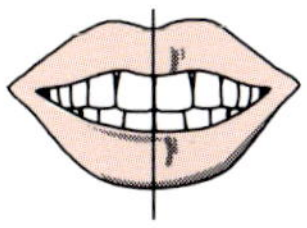

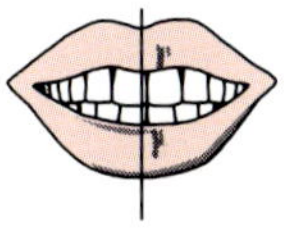

    F. Midline... Skewing to Left or Right
        ☐ Right   ☐ Left 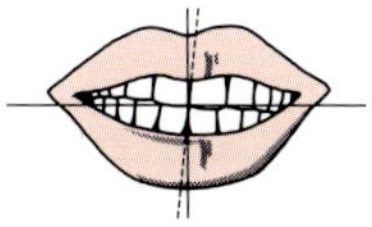   ☐ Straight

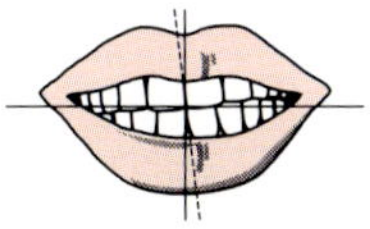

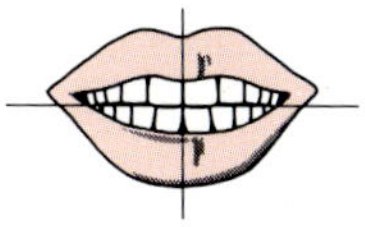

    G. Bilateral Negative Space
        ☐ Normal   ☐ Increased

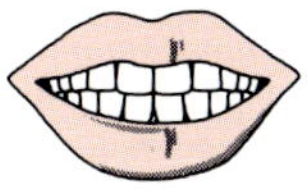

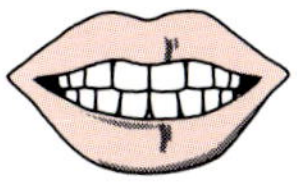

    H. Phonetics
        1. F-V sounds... Incisal edge of maxillary centrals on wet/dry line of lower lip
            ☐ Yes   ☐ No
        2. S sound... Closest speaking space—clear sound
            ☐ Yes   ☐ No

Fig. 1. The esthetic evaluation form (*continued*). The patient's smile is evaluated in a checklist form that prevents the clinician from forgetting important elements.

14 Cosmetic dentistry

4. Dental Analysis

A. Proportion of Central Incisors

Measure with calipers

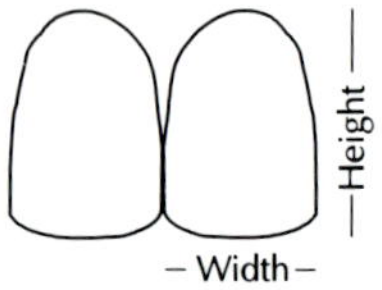

Width:Height (W:H) Ratio ☐ > 80%
☐ < 80%

The ideal Width is 80% of the Height

B. Proportion of Central to Lateral to Canine

Measure with calipers

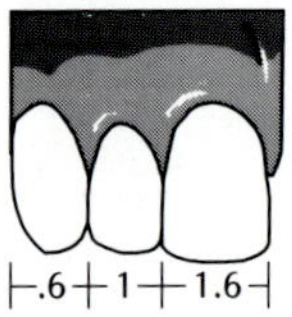

Central Width _____ mm
Lateral Width _____ mm
Cuspid Width _____ mm

.6 — 1 — 1.6

C. Axial Inclinations

Draw in Misalignment

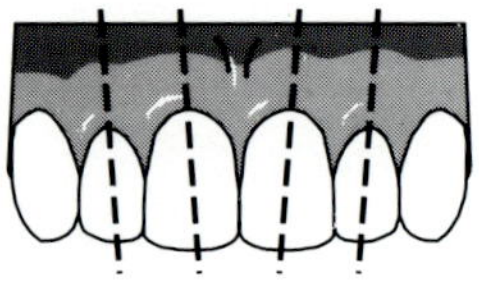

D. Gingival & Tooth Characteristics

Draw in Clinical Height of Gingiva

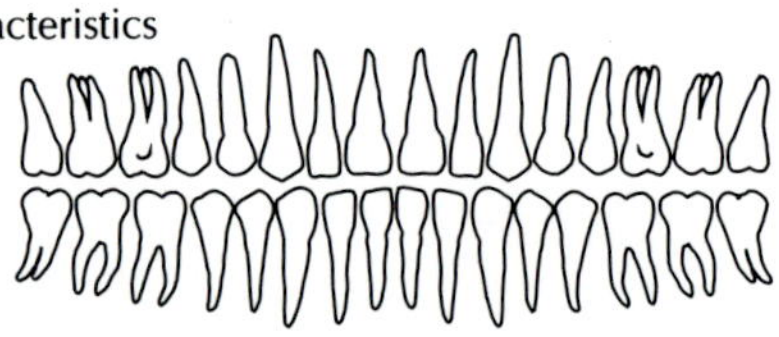

☐ Gingival Asymmetry
☐ Mucogingival Problem

5. Diagnostic Information

#	Item	Yes	No
1.	Gingival Height Symmetry — Location	☐	☐
2.	Dark Triangles — Location	☐	☐
3.	Discolored Gingiva (purple) — Location	☐	☐
4.	Overcontoured Crowns — Location	☐	☐
5.	Poor Crown Margins (open) — Location	☐	☐
6.	Active Periodontal Problems (probings) — Location	☐	☐
7.	Mobility and/or Furcation — Location	☐	☐
8.	Endodontic Lesion — Location	☐	☐
9.	Occlusion—wear facets/incisal wear — Location	☐	☐
10.	Continuous progression from canine distally (coincidence of curves) — Location	☐	☐
11.	Flared Teeth — Location	☐	☐
12.	Diastema — Location	☐	☐
13.	Overlapped Teeth — Location	☐	☐
14.	Chipped Teeth — Location	☐	☐
15.	Discolored Teeth — Location	☐	☐
16.	Surface Texture... Smooth	☐	☐

☐ Light ☐ Medium ☐ High

6. Diagnostic Information Checklist

☐ Esthetic Evaluation Form ☐ Study Casts... Diagnostic Wax-ups ☐ Computer Imaging or Similar Visualization Tool

7. Additional Notes _____

To order additional copies of the Esthetic Evaluation form, contact Pro-Dentec Canada (800) 667-3381   FAX (604) 535-7320
Copyright © 1994, Source Dental Image Inc. All rights reserved

Fig. 1. The esthetic evaluation form (*concluded*). In the dental analysis, tooth proportion and tooth-to-tooth proportion are evaluated mathematically. The diagnostic information section is a simple yes-no checklist reviewing periodontics, endodontics, and function. (*Courtesy of* Source Dental Image, Vancouver, Canada; form designed by the author.)

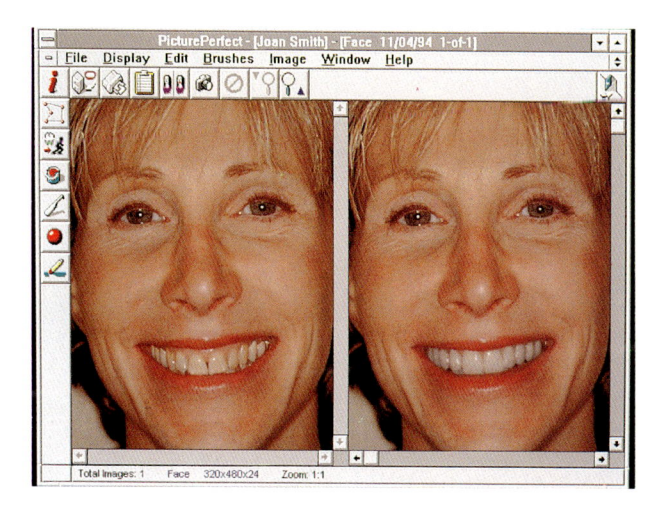

Fig. 2. An example of computer imaging. The image on the left is an unaltered "before" photograph; that on the right shows the proposed changes. With this technique, the patient's goals and expectations are revealed at the beginning of treatment, and costly remakes and failures are avoided.

3. Use the law of golden proportion for tooth-to-tooth proportion. The ratio of the widths of the central incisor, lateral incisor, and cuspid is 1.6 to 1.0 to 0.6.

4. Direct the axial inclination toward the distal.

5. Trigonal shapes of teeth, proper line angle.

6. Progression of incisal embrasures, larger as it moves from the central incisor to the cuspid, direction parallel to tooth midline.

7. Texture and incisal edge contour help create a natural look.

8. Properly position the gingival height; either remove or add pink wax to simulate proposed gingival changes. View the tissue height and relate it to the length.

The diagnostic wax-up provides a clear, three-dimensional view (Fig. 3, *right*) of the proposed changes as developed by the two-dimensional computer image.

In summary, the esthetic evaluation form is used to evaluate the smile, the face, the teeth and gingiva, and phonetics in a checklist fashion [24], assisted by the asking of effective questions. The computer imager continues the evaluation process and the search for solutions. As interaction between the parties develops, necessary changes are identified and the solutions are visualized. The diagnostic wax-up verifies the images generated by the computer.

Completing these three steps generates significant insights that ensure the success of the esthetic treatment (Figs. 4 and 5). When doctor and patient work together, communication is maximized, and a clear understanding of the patient's perception of esthetics is gained. Effective questions help build strong relationships between the patient and the dentist, allowing the patient to drive the esthetic diagnosis. If these steps are not followed, the consultation is one-sided, and the patient will lose trust in the doctor.

Conclusions

Esthetic diagnosis must be viewed in the context of improving communication between the dentist and

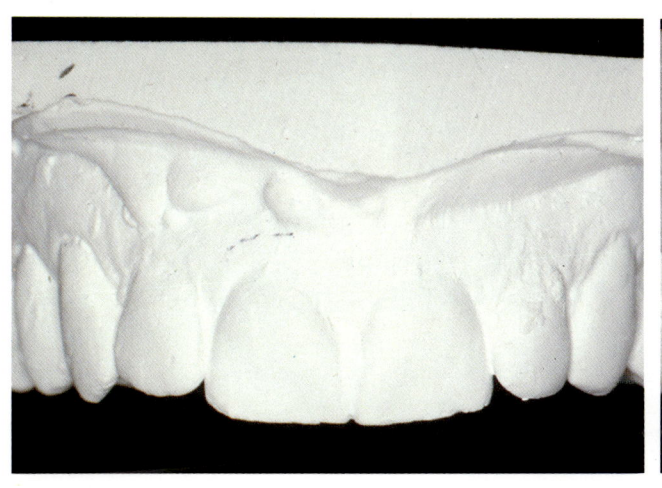

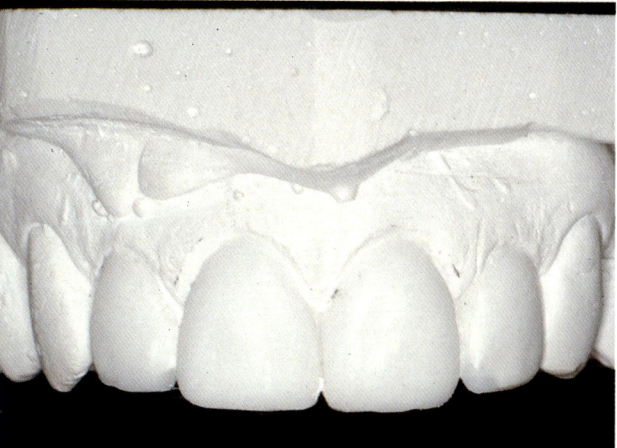

Fig. 3. The diagnostic wax-up follows the basic rules of esthetics. A preoperative diagnostic cast is taken (*left panel*), and a precise, three-dimensional blueprint of the provisional veneers is prepared (*right panel*). In turn, the provisional veneers help the technician to fabricate the final work.

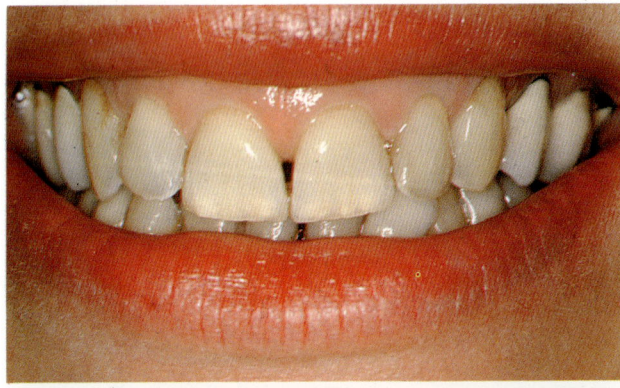

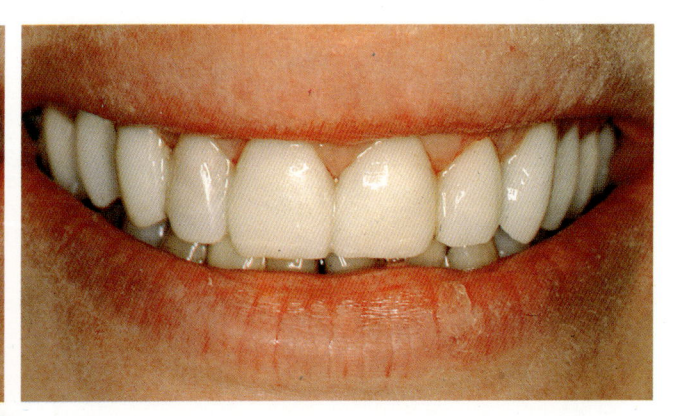

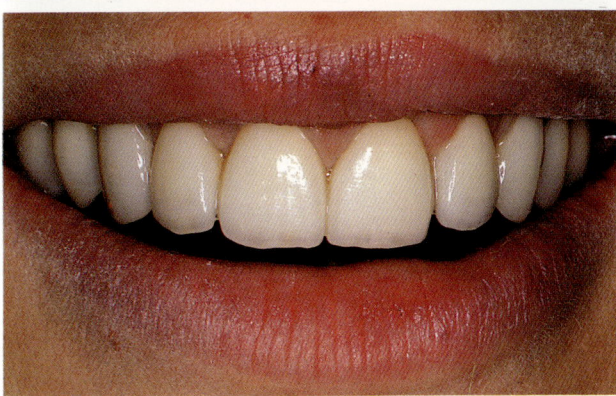

Fig. 4. Esthetic diagnosis begins with a three-step analysis of the patient's smile (*upper left panel*) that establishes the ground work for the provisional veneers (*upper right panel*). The "provisional" is the three-dimensional blueprint that guides the technician precisely to a successful final result (*bottom panel*). In this case, partial correction of the gingival area around teeth 8 and 9 was also performed, as defined by computer imaging. (*Periodontal surgery performed* by F. Celenza, New York, NY.)

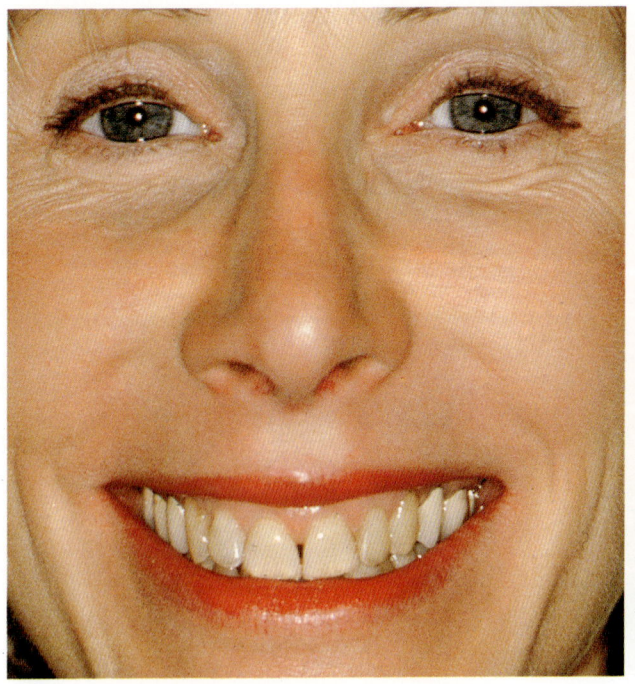

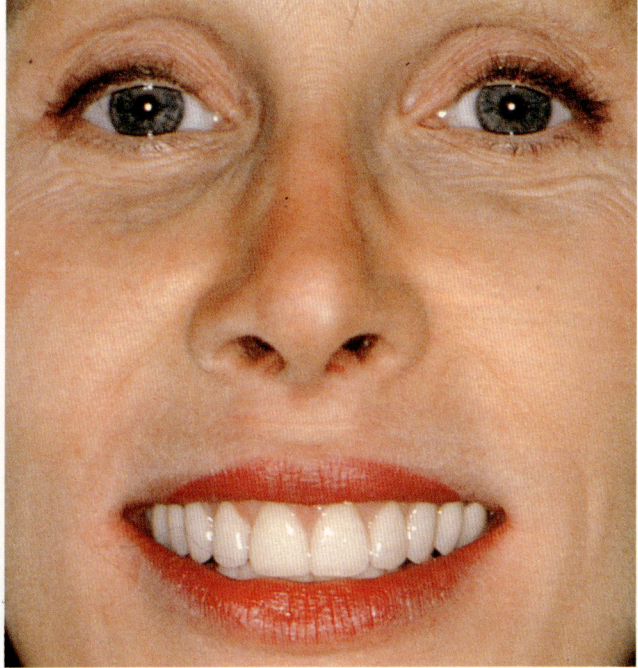

Fig. 5. Full-face views of a patient before (*left panel*) and after (*right panel*) cosmetic dentistry. A structured approach takes the clinician through a series of steps that clearly define problems and solutions.

the patient and thereby improving the understanding of the patient's concept of esthetics. What we as dentists and as individuals might consider beautiful and natural may conflict with what the patient has in mind (Miller and Lloyd, Paper presented at the International Ceramic Symposium, New Orleans, 1991). How can we know our patient's esthetic preferences if we don't ask? Effective questions must be asked, and the answers must be an important consideration in treatment development.

The structure proposed in this article incorporates a three-step analysis of esthetic treatment using comprehensive esthetic evaluation forms, computer imaging, and the diagnostic wax-up. This approach works by developing a high-energy, high-trust relationship that focuses on understanding the wants and needs of the patient and involving him or her in the decision-making process. It will serve to increase the probability of successful and consistent treatment, while improving our general understanding of esthetic concepts. In the words of the Chinese proverb, "Tell me, and I'll forget. Show me, and I may remember. Involve me, and I'll understand."

Acknowledgments

I would like to thank Dr. Jill J. DeBiasi and Dr. David Gane for their help with the esthetic evaluation form, Piera Viscido for her excellent technical work on the framework and porcelain in the clinical case, and James Washington and Beth Bay for their great assistance in the typing and editing of the manuscript.

References and recommended reading

Papers of particular interest, published within the annual period of review, have been highlighted as:
- Of special interest
- •• Of outstanding interest

1. Sheets CG: **Modern dentistry and the esthetically aware patient.** *J Am Dent Assoc* 1987, **Special issue**:103E–105E.

2. Albers H: **Esthetic treatment planning.** *Adept Report* 1992, 3:45–52.

3. Brigante RF: **Patient-assisted esthetics.** *J Prosthet Dent*, 1981, **46**:1.

4. Albino JE, Tedasco LA, Conny JD: **Patient perception of dental facial esthetics: shared concerns in orthodontics and prosthodontics** *J Prosthet Dent* 1984, **52**:9.

5. Hirsch B, Levin B, Tiber N: **Effect of patient involvement and esthetic preference or denture acceptance.** *J Prosthet Dent* 1972, **28**:127–132.

6. Brisman AS: **Esthetics: a comparison of dentists' and patients' concepts.** *J Am Dent Assoc* 1980, **100**:345.

7. Romani KL, Agahi F, Nanda R, Zernik JH: **Evaluation of**
• **horizontal and vertical differences in facial profiles by orthodontists and lay people.** *Angle Orthod* 1993, **63**:175–182.
Twenty-two clinicians and 22 lay persons completed questionnaires pertaining to their level of sensitivity to changes in facial profiles and their preferences regarding alternative profiles. Results showed that orthodontists and lay persons are sensitive to small horizontal changes in facial profile, and orthodontists are less sensitive than lay persons to large vertical changes.

8. Dawson PE: *Evaluation, Diagnosis, and Treatment of Occlusal Problems.* St. Louis: CV Mosby Co.; 1974.

9. Lombardi RA: **Method for classification of errors in dental esthetics.** *J Prosthet Dent* 1974, **32**:501–513.

10. Golub J: **Entire smile pivotal to teeth design.** *Clin Dent* 1988, **33**.

11. Chiche G, Pinault A: *Esthetics of Anterior Fixed*
•• *Prosthodontics.* Chicago: Quintessence Publishing Co.; 1994.
A great esthetic dentistry reference covering treatment planning and presenting practical advice on performing esthetic anterior restoration. Beautiful technical and color photographs throughout.

12. Rufenacht CR: *Fundamentals of Esthetics.* Chicago: Quintessence Publishing Co.; 1990.

13. Tjan A, Miller G: **Some esthetic factors in a smile.** *J Prosthet Dent*, 1984, **51**: 24–28.

14. Vig RG, Brundo GC, **The kinetics of anterior tooth display.** *J Prosthet Dent*, 1978, **39**: 502–505.

15. Allen EP: **Use of mucogingival surgical procedures to enhance esthetics.** *Dent Clin North Am* 1988, **32**:307–330.

16. Pound E: **Personalized denture procedures.** In *Dentist's Manual.* Anaheim: Denar Corp.; 1973:10.

17. Miller EL, Bodden WR, Jamison HC: **A study of the relationship of the dental midline to the facial median line.** *J Prosthet Dent*, 1979, **41**: 657–660.

18. Muia PJ: **Esthetic harmony.** In *The Four Dimensional Tooth Color System.* Chicago: Quintessence Publishing Co; 1985: 221–245.

19. Appleby DC, Craig C: **Subtleties of contour: a system for recognition and connection.** *Compendium* 1986, **7**:109–120.

20. Levin EI: **Dental esthetics and the golden proportion.** *J Prosthet Dent* 1978, **40**:244–252.

21. Oakley E, Krug D: **The ultimate empowerment tool.** In *Enlightened Leadership: Getting to the Heart of Change.* New York: Simon and Shuster; 1991:138–166.

22. Jameson C: **Presenting your recommendations effectively.** *J Am Acad Cosmetic Dent* 1991, **6**:1.

23. Levin R: **Educating the esthetic patient.** *J Am Acad Cosmetic Dent* 1992, **8**:26–27.

24. Kopp FR, Belser UC: *Esthetic Guidelines for Restorative Dentistry.* Chicago: Quintessence Publishing Co.; 1982.

Jonathan B. Levine, DMD, 923 Fifth Avenue, New York, NY 10021, USA.

Esthetic periodontics

Frank Celenza, Jr, DDS

New York University College of Dentistry, New York, New York, USA

> Periodontal therapy has developed beyond the scope of the treatment of periodontal pathoses. Periodontal plastic surgery has evolved beyond the techniques of mucogingival surgery and now consists of the regenerative and reconstructive procedures designed to enhance esthetics. This article briefly reviews the historical development of root coverage, ridge augmentation, and papilla preservation and provides an update of the current pertinent literature.

Significant advances in the field of periodontics have led to a better understanding of the biology and healing potential of the periodontal complex. This, in turn, has resulted in the evolution of treatment modalities geared toward reestablishing a more natural and cosmetic dentition. Whereas periodontal surgery has historically been considered an excisional technique, the shift toward a more reconstructive art is now well under way. The acceptance of implant dentistry as a viable treatment modality has helped to fuel some of the developments, as the demands for restoration of the dentition have progressed beyond the restoration of function. Periodontal procedures designed to enhance esthetics have come to be referred to as *periodontal plastic surgery* [1]. Periodontal plastic surgery has evolved from the original concepts and techniques of mucogingival surgery, and its scope now includes a broader range of treatment. This paper reviews the most recent advances in the techniques of root coverage, ridge augmentation, and preservation of the interdental papilla.

Root coverage

Grafting techniques have evolved to the point where both the number of procedures available and the number of applications for these procedures have increased. Previously, free gingival grafts were used for the augmentation of attached gingiva and for vestibular deepening, but now grafting of tissues, either by repositioning, transplanting, or a combination of the two, allows the surgeon to expand the application to include root coverage. Additionally, the development of guided tissue regeneration has aided in this area.

Successful root coverage can be ensured by applying the classification scheme devised by Miller [2]. Once the situation is diagnosed, the most applicable technique can be selected. Free grafts, contiguous grafts, or a combination of the two have been used with varying degrees of success in covering root surfaces of various morphologies.

Free grafts can be of two basic types, based on their source. The free gingival autograft (FGG) comes from either the palatal mucosa or other areas of adequate gingival tissue, and the subepithelial connective tissue autograft (CTG) comes from tissue lying below masticatory mucosa, usually palatally (Fig. 1). Although the surgical technique for the FGG has become relatively standardized, several techniques for the CTG have been described [3,4]. A recent study by Jahnke et al. [5•] compared the predictability in attaining root coverage of Miller class I and II marginal tissue recession defects with either FGG or CTG. Their results suggested that both techniques effectively increase the width of keratinized tissue; although the CTG may provide a greater percentage of root coverage than the FGG. Hall and Lundergan [6•] recently concurred that the FGG should not be used in areas of inadequate attached gingiva when root coverage is indicated. However, Michaelides and Wilson [7•] showed that using FGGs for root coverage was both effective and reproducible in successfully maintaining reduced gingival recession over denuded roots for a sustained period. They believed that by using different instrumentation and fewer sutures than originally proposed by Holbrook and Ochsenbein [8], surgical time could be reduced without sacrificing the quality of the result. Contiguous grafts were first introduced by Grupe and Warren [9] and became known as the *laterally positioned pedicle graft*. Whereas the laterally positioned flap can often result in excellent esthetics in terms of color match, it requires that the adjacent donor site have adequate gingiva.

Other types of contiguous grafts are also available today. The coronally positioned flap [10–15] shares the advantage of a single surgical site and can be used for multiple recessions. The semilunar coronally repositioned flap [16], which is a simplified modification of this technique, is limited by the height and thickness of

---

Abbreviations
CTG—connective tissue autograft; **FGG**—free gingival autograft.

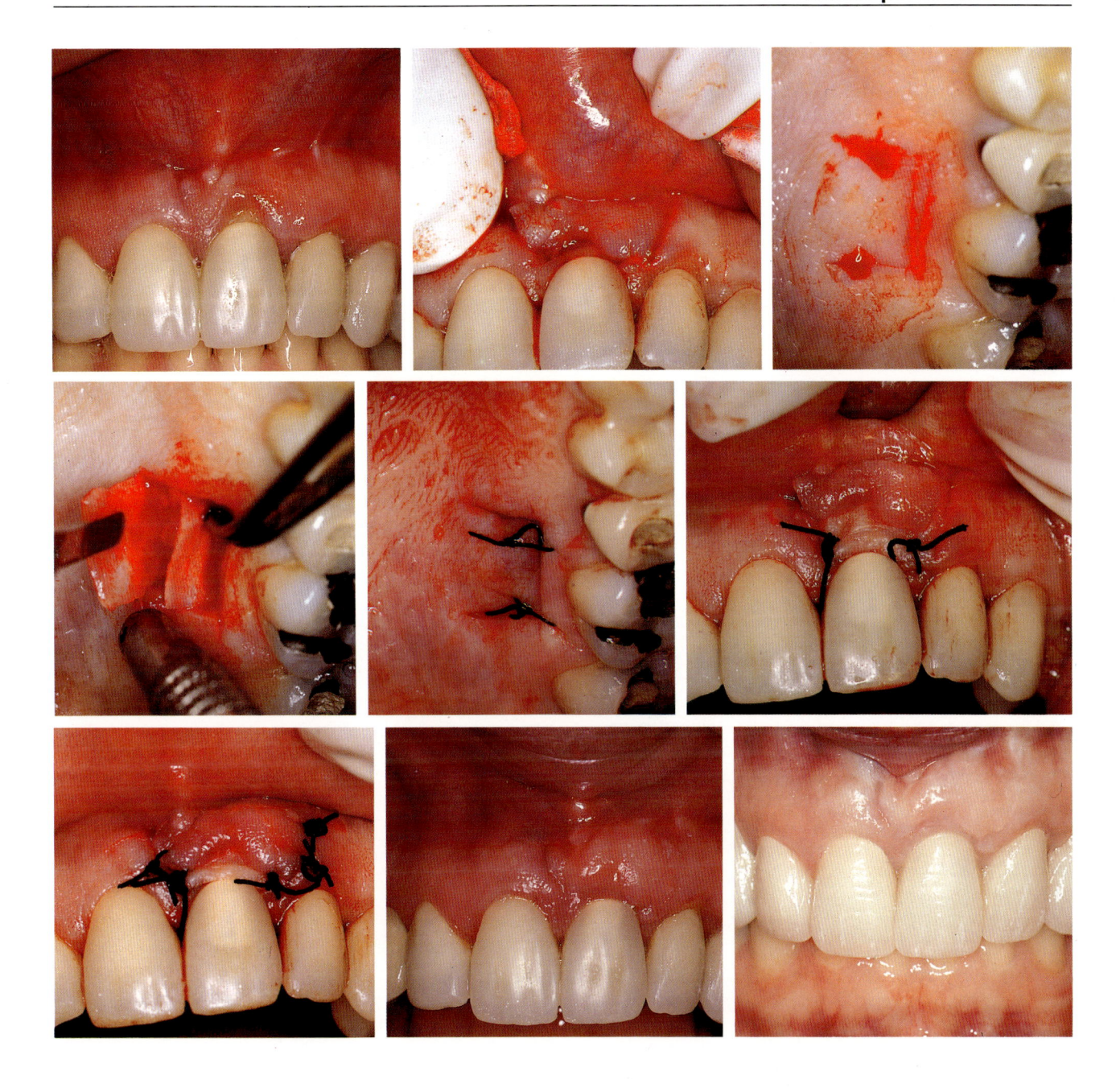

Fig. 1. **Top row left**, Recession of maxillary left central incisor in provisional stage. Esthetic restoration required even gingival margins for the central incisors. **Top row center**, Release and elevation of partial-thickness labial flap to prepare recipient site. **Top row right**, Incisions to palatal donor site. The trap door design had vertical releasing incisions and maintained epithelial border in what became the free gingival margin of the graft. **Middle row left**, Elevation of trap door and procurement of connective tissue autograft (CTG). **Middle row center**, Primary closure of donor site minimized postoperative discomfort. **Middle row right**, Placement and suturing of CTG at recipient site. **Bottom row left**, Coronal positioning and suturing of labial flap over CTG. **Bottom row center**, Four weeks after the operation, tissue was healthy and maturing, and roots were covered. **Bottom row right**, Final prosthesis. (*Prosthetic dentistry performed by* I. Gerzon, New York, NY.)

the gingival apical to the recession and is used only in a class I recession. A double lateral coronally positioned bridging flap was recently evaluated in a 5- to 8-year follow-up study [17] that concluded that although this technique could provide some assurance of longitudinal stability, the quality of the flap can be improved by the inclusion of an FGG or CTG.

Harris and Jarris [18] studied the predictability of the coronally positioned pedicle graft using butt joints and inlaid margins in conjunction with tetracycline root conditioning to treat shallow class I defects. Root coverage of 98.8% was achieved, although neither the type of attachment nor the importance of tetracycline conditioning could be determined.

20 Cosmetic dentistry

Combination techniques whereby a CTG is covered either partially or completely have also proved to be successful [4]. Bruno [19] proposed a modification to the original Langer and Langer [4] technique, which he claims is even more suitable to root coverage over wide dehiscences. His technique eliminates the vertical releasing incisions of the overlying repositioned flap, thereby maximizing the available blood supply to the underlying CTG. Allen [20] describes a technique employing a subperiosteal envelope as the recipient site. He claims his surgical modification has several advantages, such as better graft nutrition by virtue of mobilized lateral and papillary vascular supply from adjacent overlying gingiva, and preserved esthetics owing to the maintenance of papillary integrity throughout the procedure. Moreover, this technique can be employed to cover multiple recession sites.

Barrier membranes have been introduced as a means of treating marginal tissue recession [21]. The goal of this method is to attain a new attachment apparatus of connective tissue in addition to root coverage. The technique was subsequently modified to provide for a space under the barrier for more effective regeneration [22,23•]. Greater root coverage was reported with this

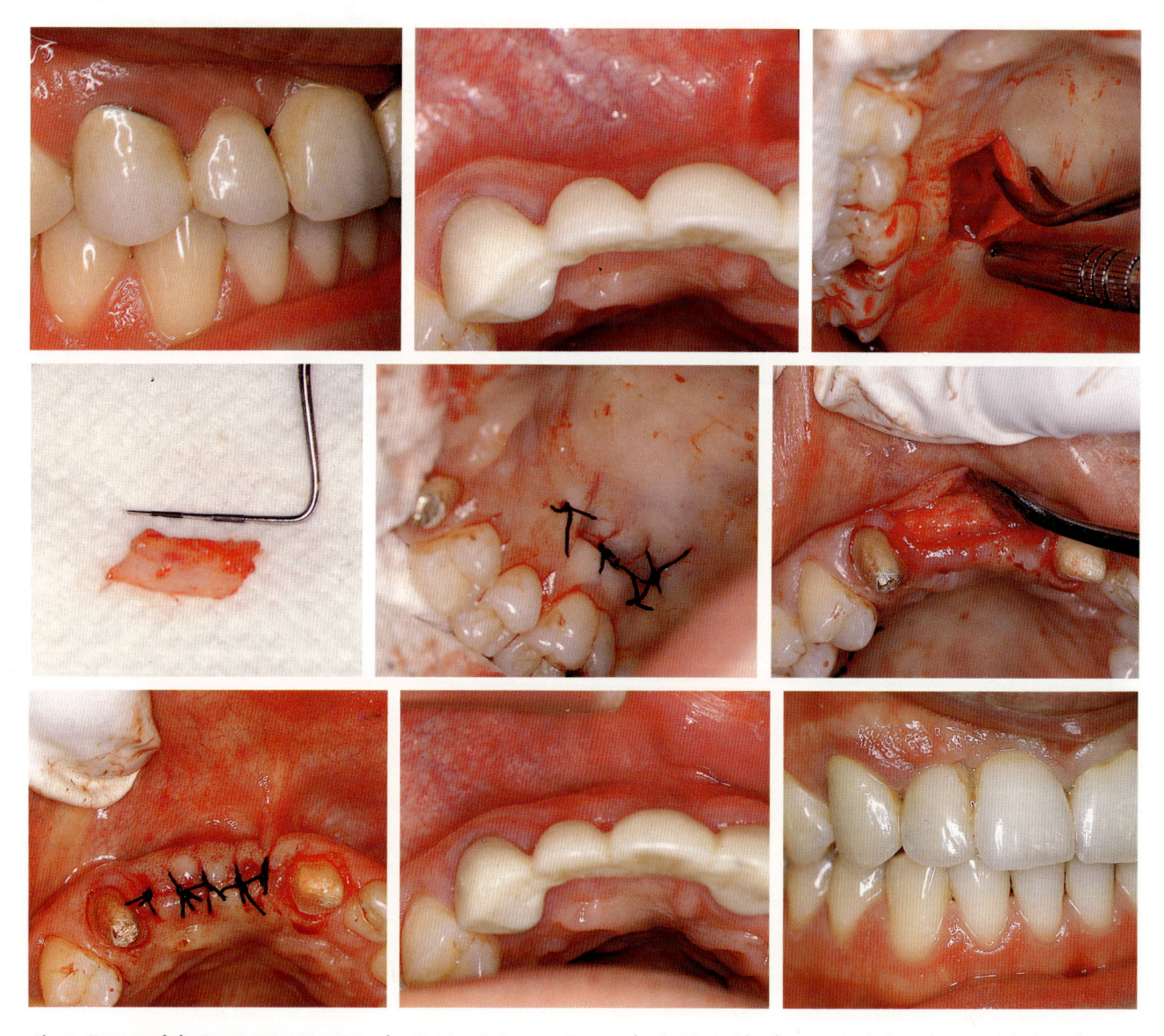

Fig. 2. Top row left, Preoperative situation of patient's existing anterior prosthesis. Note ridge lap pontic design of upper right lateral incisor necessitated by deficient ridge area. **Top row center**, Ridge concavity over maxillary right lateral incisor pontic, now in provisional prosthesis. Proper symmetry and esthetics dictated the need for ridge augmentation. **Top row right**, Trap door design to palate for harvesting of connective tissue autograft (CTG). **Middle row left**, Free CTG, in this instance without epithelial border. **Middle row center**, Primary closure of donor site. **Middle row right**, Placement of CTG into pouch preparation at recipient site. **Bottom row left**, Closure and stabilization of edentulous ridge with CTG lying subgingivally. **Bottom row center**, Four weeks after operation, added bulk to ridge over pontic was apparent. **Bottom row right**, Final prosthesis in place. Ridge augmentation allowed use of ridge lap pontic design. (*Prosthetic dentistry performed by* J. B. Levine, New York, NY.)

method. Shanaman [24•] presented two cases of the use of regeneration for root coverage. Although he offered advantages of this technique, he did not determine histologically the nature of the tooth-to-tissue interface.

Cortellini et al. [25•] performed a histologic study on a human buccal recession and demonstrated a new connective tissue attachment associated with new cementum and bone growth coronal to the previous level of the gingival margin. However, increases in the width of keratinized tissue were not addressed in any of these studies. Pini Prato et al. [26••] further developed the technique by using an FGG to cover the newly formed tissue on the root surface at reentry. In all cases, their reports showed nearly complete root coverage, which they "expect" was attached to the root surface via newly formed cementum and was further aided by the restoration of lost keratinized tissue by virtue of the FGG. Clearly, further research in this area is promising.

Ridge augmentation

Many ridge augmentation procedures are available, and they can be divided into soft-tissue mucogingival techniques, soft- or hard-tissue augmentation procedures, and soft- or hard-tissue regenerative procedures [27••]. Greater reconstructive demands placed on the edentulous ridge by the advent of implant dentistry have emphasized the need to develop these procedures. Because many ridge augmentation procedures are designed to facilitate implant placement and prosthetic function (Fig. 2), particularly with respect to hard-tissue repair, this discussion is limited to advances in soft-tissue augmentation for enhanced esthetics.

Abrams's [28] *roll technique* was one of the first soft-tissue procedures for the cosmetic improvement of a deficient pontic area. Garber and Rosenberg [29] later proposed an autogenous combined epithelial autograft and CTG. Langer and Calagna [30] applied the CTG technique to the correction of ridge deformities. Siebert [31] established a system of ridge defect classification to categorize ridge defects.

Recent developments of these techniques have been reported. Scharf and Tarnow [32••] reported on a modification of Abrams's original roll technique involving the use of a trap door to reflect and preserve overlying epithelium at the donor area. Advantages offered by this method are maximal connective tissue rolled to the buccal aspect, minimal connective tissue or bone exposure, and therefore minimal postoperative discomfort.

Wang et al. [33] demonstrated the use of connective tissue from an adjacent donor site in the form of a pedicle and its positioning beneath a partial thickness flap. Advantages offered by this method were stated to be patient comfort, improved vascularization, and more specific placement of the graft.

Siebert [34•] described the use of pouch procedures and onlay grafting. He stated that pouch-type procedures are well suited for buccolingual ridge deformities, and that onlay grafts should be employed when ridge height in an apicocoronal dimension is desired. Furthermore, the onlay graft technique requires that an abundant blood supply be available with rapid capillary proliferation. Occasionally, multiple procedures must be sequenced to achieve a desirable result.

Preservation of the interdental papilla

The treatment of maxillary anterior periodontal pathosis often requires surgical access to the root surfaces. Studies have shown that surgery performed in areas with shallow pockets can lead to recession [35–37]. The resulting cosmetic deformities in this region can be objectionable. Although nonsurgical therapy may be a suitable alternative for some cases, surgical procedures to preserve esthetics continue to be developed for more definitive therapy. Frisch et al. [38] proposed a modified resective technique aimed at conservation of maxillary anterior esthetics. Lie [39] elaborated on this technique and presented case results. The technique features soft-tissue resection along the palatal and proximal areas only, thereby granting access to the root surfaces while minimizing facial soft-tissue reflection and subsequent recession. The author noted that although the position of the facial gingival tissues remained unchanged postoperatively, a certain amount of shrinkage of the proximal papilla occurred. Nevertheless, Lie concluded that the modified resective procedures represents a simple and sometimes favorable alternative to traditional flap designs.

Whereas some surgical techniques are directed at preserving the interdental papilla, others strive to restore it. Beagle [40•] presented a case report in which a collapsed interdental papilla was surgically reconstructed. His technique combined principles of Abrams's roll technique for ridge augmentation with a papilla preservation technique proposed by Evian et al. [41], who observed an improved cosmetic result that remained stable, with only slight shrinkage, over an 18-month period.

Conclusions

Periodontal plastic surgery is constantly expanding and evolving. This trend will continue as patient and practitioner demands dictate. Soft-tissue methodologies and recent reports have been reviewed. Continued careful observation and reporting will add to the body of knowledge that will contribute to the eventual development of specific solution to an ever-expanding array of challenges.

References and recommended reading

Papers of particular interest, published within the annual period of review, have been highlighted as:
- • Of special interest
- •• Of outstanding interest

1. Miller PD: **Regenerative and reconstructive periodontal plastic surgery.** *Dent Clin North Am* 1988, 32:287–306.

2. Miller PD: **A classification of marginal tissue recession.** *J Periodontol* 1985, 2:8–13.

3. Raetzke PB: **Covering localized areas of root exposure employing the envelope technique.** *J Periodontol* 1985, 56:397–402.

4. Langer B, Langer L: **Subepithelial connective tissue graft technique for root coverage.** *J Periodontol* 1985, 60:715–720.

5. Jahnke PV, Sandifer JB, Gher ME, Gray JL, Richardson AC:
   • **Thick free gingival and connective tissue autografts for root coverage.** *J Periodontol* 1993, 64:315–322.
   This paper provides a scientific comparison of the CTG and FGG methods of root coverage in Miller class I and II marginal tissue recession defects. Both techniques resulted in improved keratinized tissue and probing attachment levels, but the results suggest that whereas both techniques can effectively increase the width of keratinized tissue, the CTG may provide a higher percentage of root coverage.

6. Hall WB, Lundergan WP: **Free gingival grafts: current indica-**
   • **tions and techniques.** *Dent Clin North Am* 1993, 37:227–242.
   An up-to-date description of the indications and contraindications for the use of FGGs in light of the introduction of more advanced techniques. More specifically, the paper states that the FGG is an appropriate procedure to augment an inadequate band of attached gingiva, if esthetics is not a primary concern and root coverage is not an objective.

7. Michaelides PL, Wilson SG: **An autogenous gingival graft**
   • **technique.** *Int J Periodontics Restorative Dent* 1994, 14:113–125.
   The authors describe and modify the FGG technique for root coverage and observe the stability of the results.

8. Holbrook T, Ochsenbein C: **Complete coverage of denuded root surfaces with a one-stage gingival graft.** *Int J Periodontics Restorative Dent* 1983, 3:9–27.

9. Grupe HE, Warren RF: **Repair of gingival defects by a sliding flap operation.** *J Periodontol* 1956, 27:290–295.

10. Allen EP, Miller PD: **Coronal positioning of existing gingiva: short-term results in the treatment of shallow marginal tissue recession.** *J Periodontol* 1989, 66:316–319.

11. Nordenram A: **Parodontalkirurgish Rekonstruktion av gingival Rander erter Gingivektomi same Seans.** *Svensk Tandlak T* 1959, 52:173–179.

12. Harvey PM: **Management of advanced periodontitis: 1. Preliminary report of a surgical reconstruction.** *N Z Dent J* 1965, 61:180–187.

13. Nordenram A, Landt A: **Evaluation of a surgical technique in the periodontal treatment of maxillary anterior teeth.** *Acta Odontol Scand* 1969, 27:283–289.

14. Restrepo OJ: **Coronally repositioned flap: report of 4 cases.** *J Periodontol* 1973, 44:564–567.

15. Caffesse RG, Guinard EA: **Treatment of localized gingival recessions: part II. Coronal repositioned flap in periodontal therapy.** *J Periodontol* 1978, 49:357–361.

16. Tarnow DP: **Semilunar coronally positioned flap.** *J Clin Periodontol* 1986, 13:182–185.

17. Romanos GE, Bernimoulin JP, Marggraf E: **The double lateral bridging flap for coverage of denuded root surface: longitudinal study and clinical evaluation after 5 to 8 years.** *J Periodontol* 1993, 64:683–688.

18. Harris RJ, Jarris AW: **The coronally positioned pedicle graft with inlaid margins: a predictable method of obtaining root coverage of shallow defects.** *Int J Periodontics Restorative Dent* 1994, 25:229–241.

19. Bruno JP: **Connective tissue graft technique assuring wide root coverage.** *Int J Periodontics Restorative Dent* 1994, 14:127–137.

20. Allen AL: **Use of the supraperiosteal envelope in soft tissue grafting for root coverage: I. Rationale and technique.** *Int J Periodontics Restorative Dent* 1994, 14:217–227.

21. Tinti C, Vincenzi G, Cortellini P, Pini Prato G, Clauser C: **Guided tissue regeneration in the treatment of human facial recession: a 12-case report.** *J Periodontol* 1992, 63:554–560.

22. Pini Prato GP, Tinti C, Vincenzi G, Magnani C, Cortellini P, Clauser C: **Guided tissue regeneration versus mucogingival surgery in the treatment of human buccal recession.** *J Periodontol* 1992, 63:919–928.

23. Tinti C, Vincenzi G, Cocchetto R: **Guided tissue regeneration**
    • **in mucogingival surgery.** *J Periodontol* 1993, 64:1184–1191.
    The authors describe the use of guided tissue regeneration to correct mucogingival problems, specifically recession. A trapezoidal flap design and a modified suturing technique are employed in an attempt to create a place under the membrane. This technique may be the precursor to the titanium-reinforced membranes that are now available.

24. Shanaman RH: **Gingival augmentation using guided tissue**
    • **regeneration: two case reports.** *Int J Periodontics Restorative Dent* 1993, 13:373–377.
    This paper points up a number of advantages of the use of guided tissue regeneration over conventional root coverage procedures and presents two case reports.

25. Cortellini P, Clauser C, Pini Prato GO: **Histologic assessment**
    • **of new attachment following the treatment of a human buccal recession by means of a guided tissue regeneration procedure.** *J Periodontol* 1993, 64:387–391.
    This paper is the first published report of the histologic findings in the treatment of a human buccal recession applying the guided tissue regeneration method. New connective tissue attachment with newly formed cementum and bone growth is demonstrated. Posttreatment crestal bone levels are found crestal to the preoperative location of the gingival margin.

26. Pini Prato G, Clauser C, Cortellini P: **Guided tissue regenera-**
    •• **tion and a free gingival graft for the management of buccal recession: a case report.** *Int J Periodontics Restorative Dent* 1993, 13:487–493.
    This paper describes the use of guided tissue regeneration to achieve a new attachment and an FGG to augment the zone of keratinized gingiva over the newly formed tissue on the root surface. Theoretically, this would result in the complete reconstruction of a damaged periodontium. The use of the FGG has the additional advantage of restoring the mucogingival junction to its original position, thereby preventing vestibular shallowing.

27. Rosenberg ES, Cutler SA: **Periodontal considerations for es-**
    •• **thetics: edentulous ridge augmentation.** *Curr Opin Cosmetic Dent* 1993, 1:61–66.
    This paper provides an excellent review and classification of the many ridge augmentation procedures. Therapy is divided into soft-tissue mucogingival techniques, soft- or hard-tissue augmentation procedures, and soft- or hard-tissue regenerative procedures.

28. Abrams L: **Augmentation of the deformed residual edentulous ridge for fixed prostheses.** *Compendium* 1980, 1:205–214.

29. Garber DA, Rosenberg ES: **The edentulous ridge in fixed prosthodontics.** *Compendium* 1981, 2:212–223.

30. Langer B, Calagna L: **The subepithelial connective tissue graft.** *J Prosthet Dent* 1980, 44:363–367.

31. Siebert SJ: **Reconstruction of deformed partially edentulous ridges using full thickness onlay grafts: part II. Prosthetic/periodontal interrelationships.** *Compendium* 1983, 4:549–562.

32. Scharf DR, Tarnow DP: **Modified roll technique for localized alveolar ridge augmentation.** *Int J Periodontics Restorative Dent* 1992, 12:415–425.
••
This paper describes a modification to the Abrams's original roll technique for ridge augmentation (*Compendium* 1980, 1:205–214). Advantages of the technique are described, and two cases are presented with diagrams that clearly illustrate the method. By preserving the overlying palatal epithelium rather than resecting it, it is believed, the technique offers the advantages of reducing patient discomfort and maximizing the amount of connective tissue that can be rolled into the augmentation site.

33. Wang PD, Pitman DP, Jans HH: **Ridge augmentation using a subepithelial connective tissue pedicle graft.** *Pract Periodontics Aesthet Dent* 1993, 5:47–51.

34. Siebert JS: **Reconstruction of the partially edentulous ridge: gateway to improved prosthetics and superior aesthetics.** *Pract Periodontics Aesthet Dent* 1993, 5:47–55.
•
A review and discussion of the two types of soft-tissue ridge augmentations—pouch procedures and onlay grafts.

35. Pihlstrom BL, Ortiz-Campos C, McHugh RB: **A randomized four-year study of periodontal therapy.** *J Periodontol* 1981, 52:227.

36. Knowles JW, Burgett FG, Nissle RR, *et al.*: **Results of periodontal treatment related to pocket depth and attachment level. Eight years** *J Periodontol* 1979, 50:225.

37. Ramfjord SP, Caffesse RG, Morrison EC, *et al.*: **Four modalities of periodontal treatment compared over 5 years.** *J Clin Periodontol* 1987, 14:445.

38. Frisch J, Jones RA, Bhaskar SN: **Conservation of maxillary anterior esthetics: a modified surgical approach.** *J Periodontol* 1967, 38:11.

39. Lie T: **Periodontal surgery for the maxillary anterior area.** *Int J Periodontics Restorative Dent* 1992, 12:73–82.

40. Beagle JR: **Surgical reconstruction of the interdental papilla: case report.** *Int J Periodontics Restorative Dent* 1992, 12:145–151.
•
The author provides diagrams and a case report to describe clearly the reconstruction of a collapsed interdental papilla. The proposed technique involves a combination of the Abrams's original roll technique for ridge augmentation (*Compendium* 1980, 1:205–214) with Evian's method for papilla preservation (*Compendium* 1985, 6:58–64).

41. Evian CI, Corn H, Rosenberg ES: **Retained interdental papilla procedure for maintaining anterior esthetics.** *Compendium* 1985, 6:58–64.

Frank Celenza, Jr., DDS, 532 Park Avenue, New York, NY 10021, USA.

Anterior esthetics and the visual arts: beauty, elements of composition, and their clinical application to dentistry

Thomas S. Valo, DDS

Sylvania, Ohio, USA

The challenge of developing a pleasing smile is an artistic venture. A study of how the visual arts have explored the nature of beauty and the elements of artistic composition will enhance our artistic abilities in cosmetic dentistry. This review discusses the perception of beauty and important features of that which we call beautiful. The discussion uses important works of art to demonstrate elements of composition, which are then made relevant in a dental application.

Creating high-quality, tooth-colored, tooth-shaped restorations is a challenge, but to be a cosmetic dentist, one must aspire to an even higher plane. Our goal is not merely to deliver invisible restorations but to create beautiful artistic expressions, to change a smile so that its lines and textures carry a message and enhance a face. The word *esthetic*, which we use so often in our field, refers to an understanding of beauty. We must therefore have an understanding of beauty and the artistic tools available to develop a beautiful smile.

Dentistry has considered the need for individual and artistic expression in its work since the 1950s, when individual characterizations were proposed for dentures according to the patient's phonetics, lip line, age, sex, and personality [1–8]. The importance of such an interest in creating attractive smiles is underscored by studies showing the psychosocial difficulties [9] and prejudices [10] associated with facial malformations. Conversely, physical attractiveness has value in our society in settings ranging from the classroom and job interviews [11] to making friends and dating [12•]. The oral region is of primary importance in determining overall facial attractiveness [13], surpassing even complexion, eyes, hairstyle, face shape, and nose [12•]. Recent publications reviewed the visual arts, beauty, artistic composition, and the application of artistic principles to dentistry in an effort to create more attractive or dramatic smiles [14,15•,16–19]. Similar interest has been expressed in the field of plastic surgery [20•]. A study of artistic principles should enable the clinician to create a smile that is both pleasing to the eye and satisfying to the patient.

When we look upon an object, whether it is a face, a landscape, or a painting, we begin to analyze it. Our eye is attracted first to one place in the composition, most likely the most dominant, bright, or moving part. In a face (Fig. 1), the smile contains contrasts of bright teeth against red lips and is active in speech and expression. Thus, it is dominant and attracts our attention first. When we are satisfied with our evaluation of this first area, our eye begins to follow visual channels to other less dominant parts of the face in an orderly fashion. An artist plans these visual channels in his composition using line, contrast, and the size of objects. A dentist can plan these visual channels, too, by attending to the many details of a smile, including tooth positioning, effective use of negative space in the buccal corridor, and the development of the smile line. These parts, or elements, and their relation to one another create a perception of tension or peace, serenity or vitality. It is the skilled manipulation of these parts and their resulting effect that makes for great art and great cosmetic dentistry. In cosmetic dentistry, beauty might be a desired trait in the completed smile. In theatrical dentistry, the goal might be to achieve a number of other qualities, including grotesque or absurd features. In all of dentistry, a desired effect may be accomplished through the skillful use of artistic principles.

Beauty

St. Thomas Aquinas said, "Beauty is that which, being seen, pleases." Efforts to define and capture the essence of beauty have eluded man since the beginning of history. Yet, throughout time and cultures, certain personality traits of beauty remain constant [21].

Culture

In every culture, art is found in the purely decorative, such as paintings or statues, and in practical objects, such as pottery and buildings. Artistic expression tells us about a people's spiritual beliefs, the values of their society, their perceptions of life, and their ideals of beauty. As we shall see, a cultural expression of beauty may be found in dentistry as well as in pottery and statues. To the ancient Greeks, beauty arose from a philosophy of life that exalted human values and saw their gods as nothing but men made large. Their artistic works used ideal types of humanity—perfectly formed, perfectly proportioned, noble, and serene (Fig.

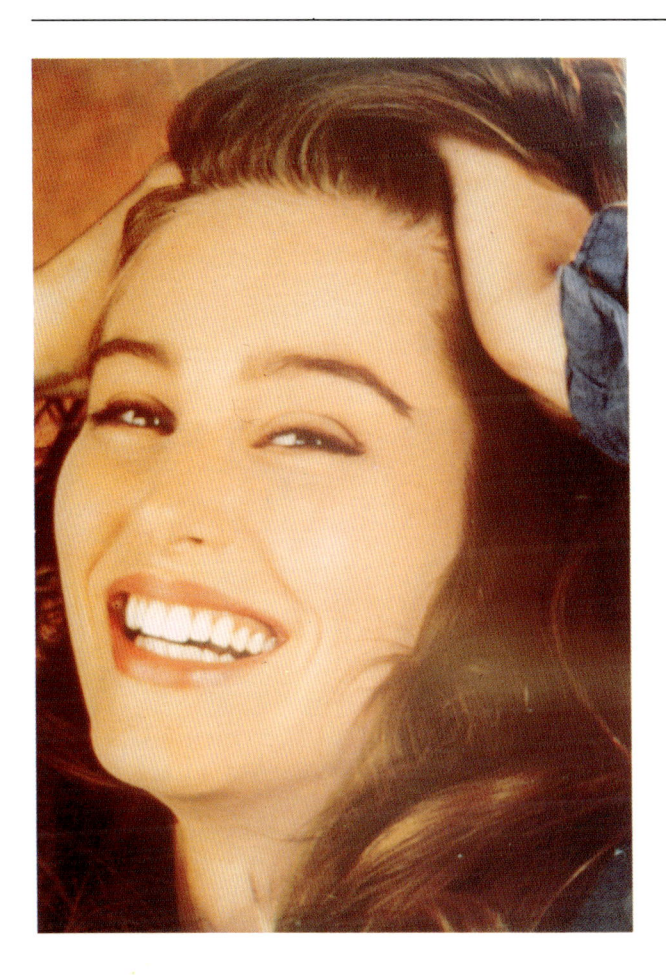

Fig. 1. Our eye is attracted first to the smile, then to less dominant parts of the face. (*From* Ultradent Products, Salt Lake City, UT; with permission.)

2) [22]. The geometric rules of Pythagoras' golden section and Plato's beautiful proportion demonstrate a desire to find a rational, physically measurable definition of beauty. This type of idealized beauty, inherited by Rome and revived at the Renaissance, is part of today's humanism. In all of these periods, spiritual thought and perceptions of life have exalted human beings, and the resulting perception of beauty focuses on physical perfection. Perhaps the perfect, unblemished white smile desired by many today belongs to this concept of beauty.

By contrast, the Byzantine era and early Christian art focused their ideals upon the divine instead of the human. The emphasis was on the intellectual and abstract instead of the physical. As a result, the artists of this period saw beauty in higher things and exalted their Creator instead of themselves (Fig. 2, *top right*). Today, some of our patients object to eliminating stains and wear from their teeth, because they feel it looks unnatural or inappropriate. They see that the rigors of life may leave signs of wear and tear, but that virtue is gained through the process of life. This value upon character and lack of concern for unblemished appearance might be likened to the concept of beauty in the Byzantine era.

A third view of beauty may be found in Oriental culture. Here the focus is on the metaphysical, explaining reality and knowledge in an instinctive intellectual manner. Oriental beauty tries to understand the mystery of a thing and does not try to imitate nature or flatter humanity (Fig. 2, *bottom left*). Through the use of color and repetitive rhythm, Oriental artists achieve great vitality, but at the expense of accurate reproduction. The Japanese geishas' practice of coloring their teeth black might be seen as beautiful to those who see beauty through a metaphysical eye (Fig. 2, *bottom right*).

All of this is meant to show that the perception of beauty varies according to culture and a perception of life. Similar expressions are found in dentistry.

Intuition

Intuition is the second personality trait of beauty. Intuition is concerned with something beyond knowledge, enjoyment. When we add preference to fact, we begin to have beauty [21]. The use of strict rules for the design of a smile, whether they are the golden proportion or development of a perfect smile line, can be only a part of the plan. It is with our intuition that we incorporate appropriate variations from the ideal to create artistically a beautiful smile.

"It should always be remembered," wrote Read [22], "that the appeal of art is not to conscious perception at all, but to intuitive apprehension. A work of art is not present in thought, but in feeling. It is a symbol rather than a direct statement of truth."

Distortion

A moralist of the Renaissance said, "There is no excellent beauty that hath not some strangeness in proportion," (quoted by Read [22]). Rather than create an exact reproduction, an artist takes his subject, then emphasizes or distorts to make a statement or express an emotion (Fig. 3). Within the bounds of physiology and function, we must be free to distort in order to create the desired illusion or impression (Fig. 4).

Variety

Variety is critical to visual beauty and interest. Visual beauty is like beautiful music or beautiful poetry. In verse, a perfectly regular meter is so monotonous as to become intolerable. Poets have therefore taken liberty with their measure; feet are reversed within the meter, and the whole rhythm counterpoised [22]. Likewise, in the visual arts and in dentistry, exact dimension may be altered to a subtle degree. The variation is not determined by laws but by the instinct and sensibility of the artist. Without variety we have monotony, but with it our interest is captured, and the potential for beauty is born.

Association

A powerful visual tool in the arts makes use of association. Classic images, such as the horse, immediately speak power and speed to the viewer. The winged

26 Cosmetic dentistry

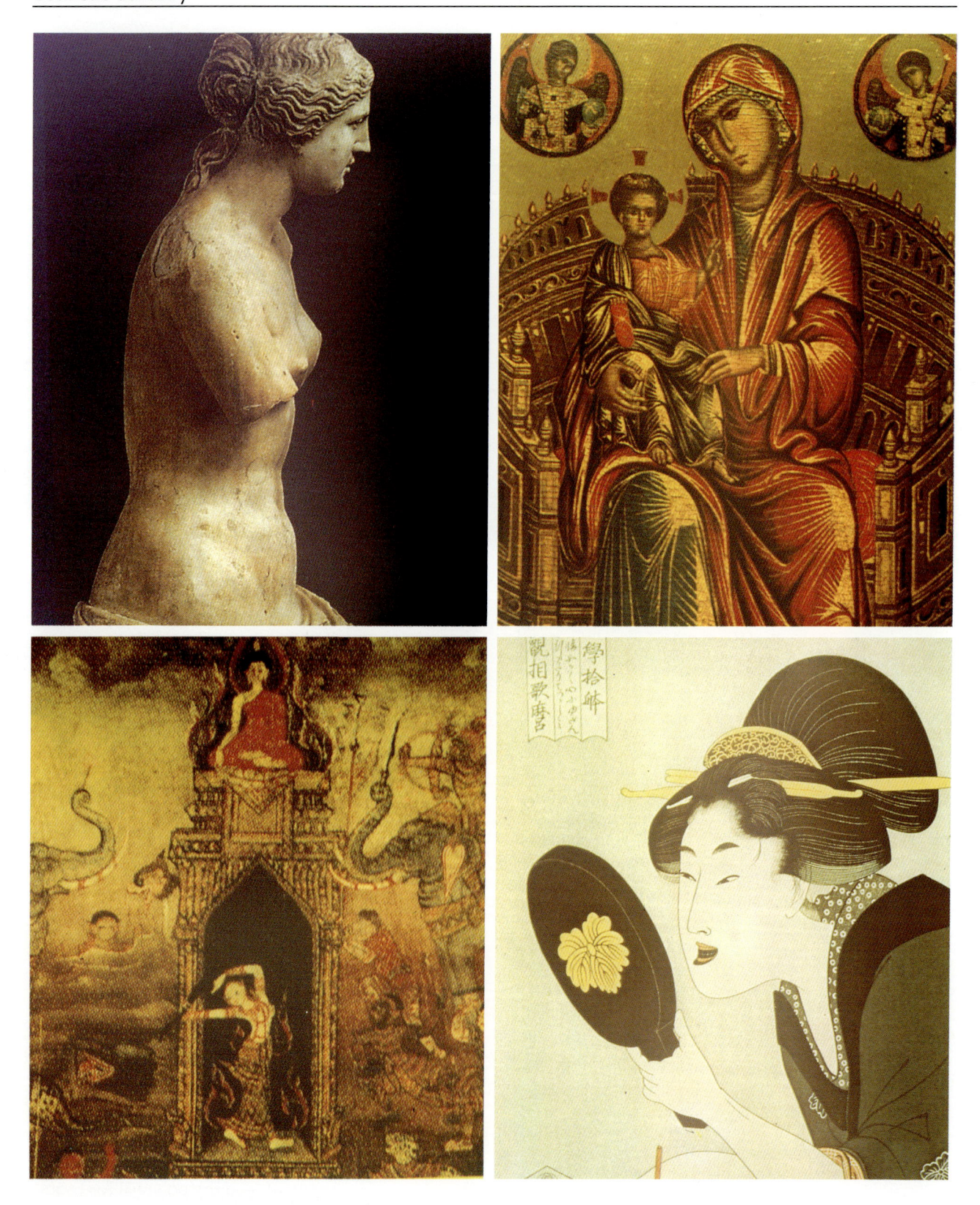

Fig. 2. Top left, The Venus of Milo, with its perfect proportion and rounded line, is a classic expression of Greek beauty. **Top right**, Early Christian art emphasized a spiritual message at the expense of physical beauty, yet these works are considered beautiful because of the meaning and emotions they depict. **Bottom left**, Color and repetitive rhythm bring out vitality in this Oriental work, rather than accurately reproducing its subject. **Bottom right**, A geisha admiring her beautiful, blackened teeth.

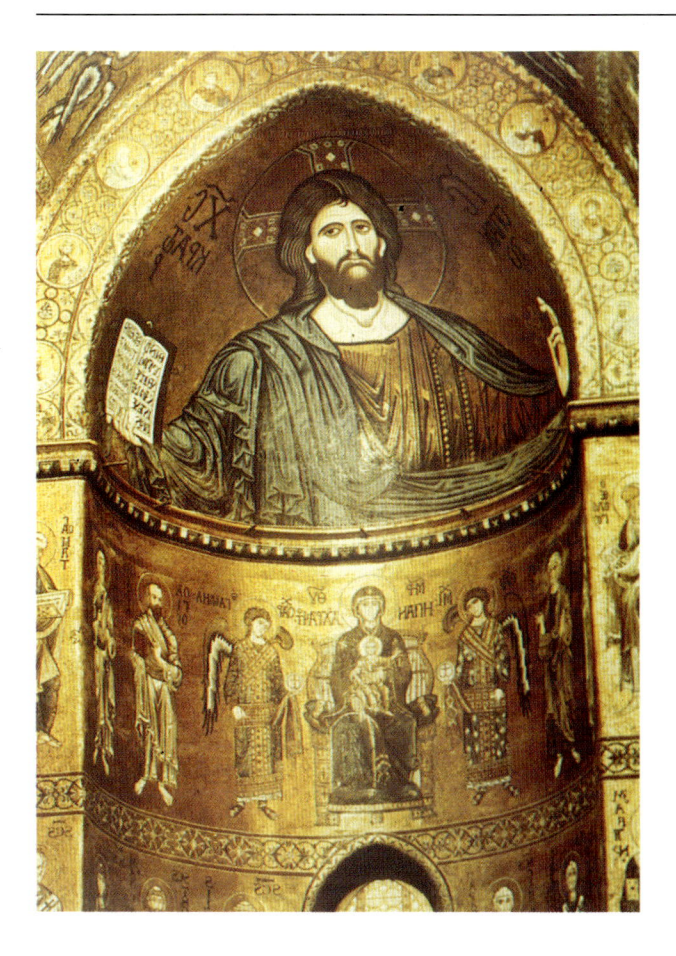

Fig. 3. Distortions used in this Byzantine altar cause us to sense awe and grandeur in the subject.

horse connotes even greater speed [22]. In cosmetic dentistry we must be aware of the power of association; emotions are quickly drawn upon when we view broken teeth (poverty, ill health), unworn teeth (youth, innocence), and a classic American beauty's smile (young adulthood, wealth, beauty) (Fig. 5).

So beauty is that pleasant experience seen with subjective senses, interpreted by our associations, filtered by a philosophy of life, capturing our imagination through variety and distortion, and felt by intuition. The essence of beauty has been sought since the beginning of time.

Subject, unity, and content

An artist's subject is simply the object with which he or she works, for example a bowl of fruit or a woman's face. The subject is not important of itself, but is merely a stimulus to creativity. The artist then uses various visual devices to present elements of the subject in such a manner as to suggest emotion or intellectual meaning. Great artists are recognized for their efficient use of all the component parts of the subject. The total effect is said to exhibit unity when everything fits, when the work has meaning. The effect is expressed clearly with a sense of oneness and without confusion (Fig. 6). This message is what is called the content of the work.

A painter uses a wide variety of subjects. A cosmetic dentist's subject is limited to teeth, gingiva, lips, and people. Like the painter, we can use visual devices in a carefully organized manner to create a desired effect. We present our work best when everything fits, and our desired effect is expressed clearly with a sense of oneness. Meaning is the common goal of the artist on canvas as well as the dentist. Is not a lasting impression, the effect of a meaningful smile, what we are after? Our study of what artists call *principles of organization* will help us to achieve this artistic result, which is what our patients want.

Principles of organization

Visual forming (ordering)
The overall effect in a work of art does not occur by accident. Rather, it is the result of painstaking planning. For example, Rembrandt's "Presentation of Christ" de-

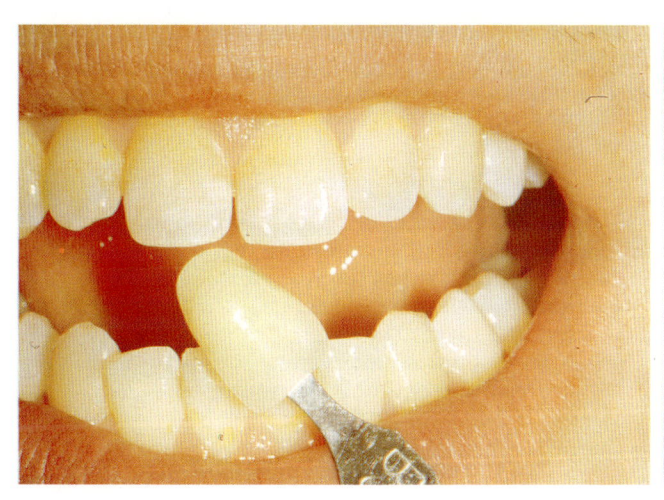

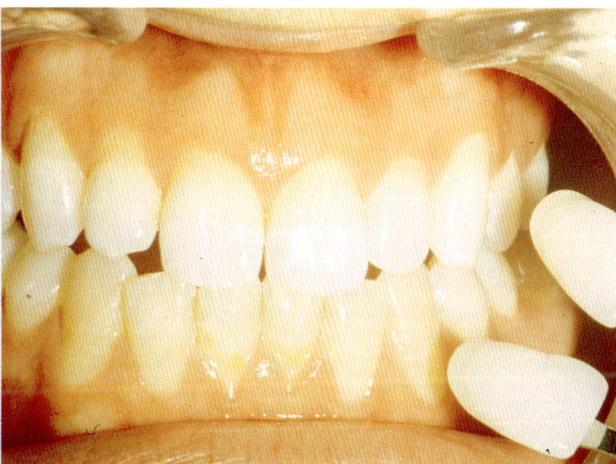

Fig. 4. Whitening of teeth distorts the original appearance of the subject and by eliminating stains utilizes the principle of economy. **Left**, Before whitening. **Right**, After whitening.

28 Cosmetic dentistry

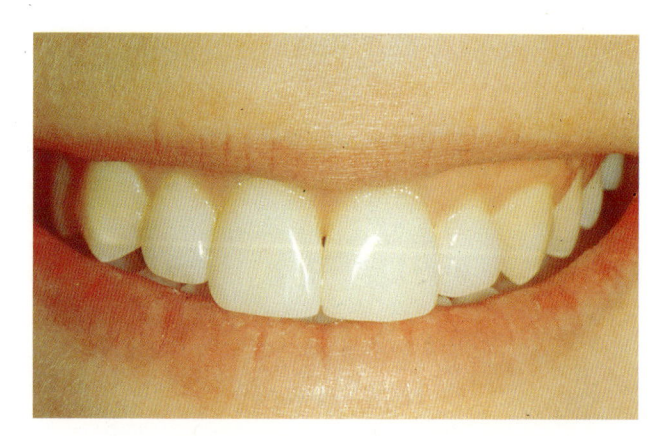

Fig. 5. Top left, This diseased smile gives its owner a look of poverty and speaks of a hard life. **Top right**, The lines in this smile are easily recognized as belonging to a young person with a quality of innocence. **Bottom**, The typical lines of an ideal smile are associated with wealth, beauty, and young adulthood.

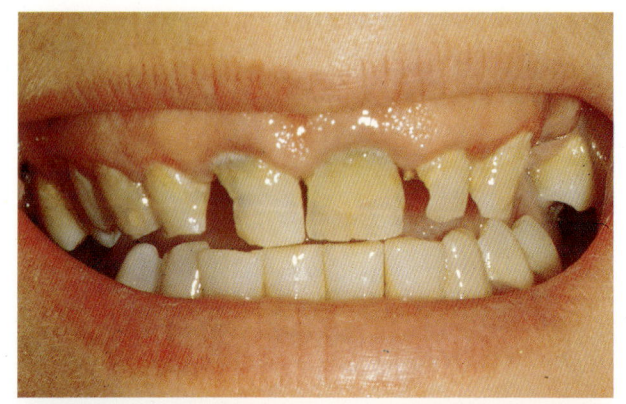

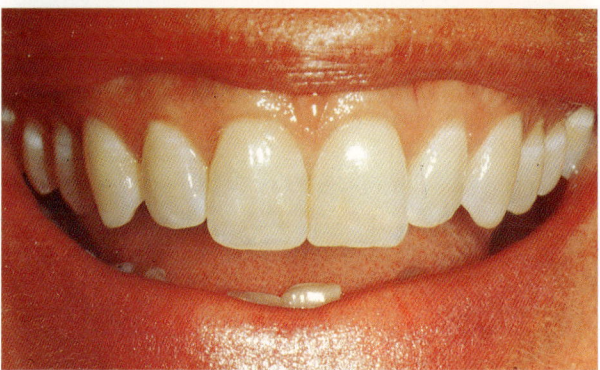

veloped out of a series of detailed sketches involving dramatic deletions and changes (Fig. 7). These were done to achieve the most interesting and communicative presentation. Rembrandt understood that our eye and mind organize various components of a picture into a unified whole, trying to create order out of chaos. He understood that our eye is attracted to bold and dominant elements first, and then drawn along visual channels through the entire work, following lines of color and texture in carefully planned order (Fig. 8). The composition reads like a chapter in a book. In visual art, the road map for the eye may be less obvious than for the written word, but it is always present.

Curiously, once this principle of visual forming is understood, it becomes evident in a smile as well. In the following paragraphs, concepts such as harmony and variety, balance, dominance, and economy are discussed. All of them are relevant to visual order. When an element is used inappropriately, the resulting smile lacks the personality that may be desired. The result instead may be confusion or a feeling that something is wrong with the smile composition.

Harmony and variety

Harmony is what holds contrasts together. It is developed with rhythm and repetition. That is, the repetition of lines, colors, shapes, and textures creates harmony. These repetitions, called rhythm, have been likened to a tempo or beat in music. They hold the composition together just as tempo, rhythm, or repeating chord progressions in music can provide continuity throughout a song. Skillful use of rhythm and repetition, with alternating pauses and beats, causes a flow or connection between parts of the work, directing eye movement from one element of the composition to another.

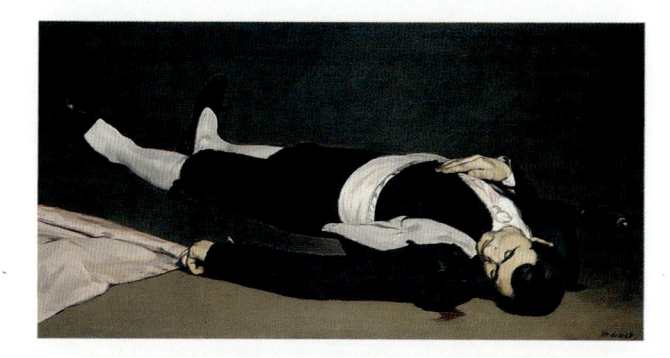

Fig. 6. A demonstration of the efficient use of all the component parts of the subject to create a clear effect. (Manet, "The Dead Toreador," Widener Collection, ©1995 Board of Trustees, National Gallery of Art, Washington, DC.)

Just as an unvaried chord progression is monotonous, so is a painting that lacks variety. Variety is introduced by increasing contrast in line, texture, color, value, and form, but variety alone is chaos without meaning. While harmony provides stability and continuity, variety captures our interest. Variety is the counterweight to harmony. The two belong together.

Now let us consider a dental application (Fig. 9). We know that the smile is the single most impressive aspect of a face. It captures another's attention, and its design is critical to beauty. There are repeating lines in a beautiful smile. The incisal edges of the upper teeth

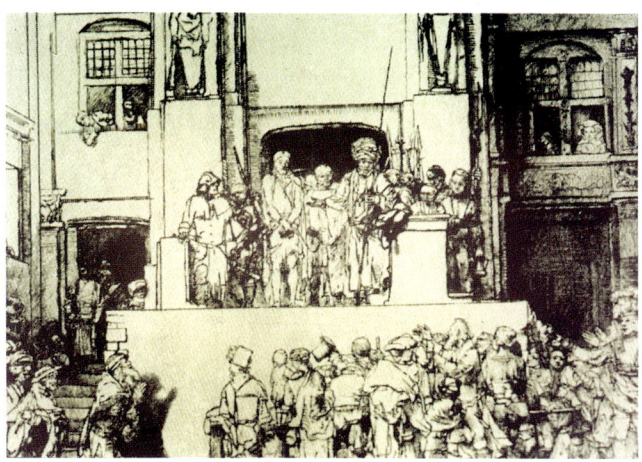

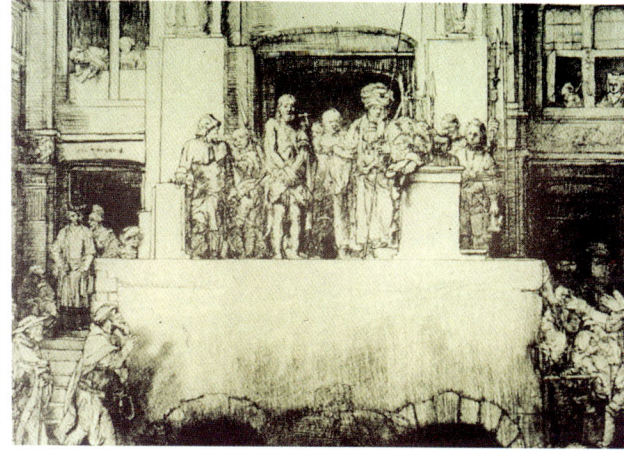

Fig. 7. In "Christ Presented to the People," Rembrandt went to great effort to work and rework his composition at least six times to achieve the most dramatic and communicative effect. In dentistry, our planning and attention to detail are also part of creating the optimum result. (The Metropolitan Museum of Art, New York, NY, gift of Felix M. Warburg and his family, 1941; used with permission.)

and the border of the lower lip form repeating lines we refer to as the smile line. This repetition imparts harmony and unity to the smile. So, too, do the repetition of vertical lines separating each tooth and the parallelism of the upper gingival line and lower border of the upper lip. On the other hand, recall the denture design referred to early in our dental careers as "Chiclet teeth." This classic denture look is simply one of monotony: uniform color, shape, and arrangement. Think of some entertainment personalities whose teeth have been the topic of common conversation due to their uniform whiteness and mechanically perfect arrangement. All of these straight white teeth have failed to compliment the owner's smile at the expense of beauty. They lack variety. Variety is incorporated by subtly varying color within each tooth and between teeth. A varied arrangement might include subtle rotations and the positioning of teeth out of the ideal. The variations that can be incorporated into a smile are endless. But beware. Just as excessive repetition creates boredom, excessive variety in tooth arrangement creates chaos at the expense of harmony.

Balance

Balance refers to the felt optical equilibrium in a composition (Fig. 10). As the eye travels over a picture, it pauses momentarily at significant parts. These parts represent moving and directional forces that must counterbalance one another, so that controlled tension results. Unbalanced artwork looks unfinished, accidental, and full of tension. When the work is balanced, the tension is released. Similarly, when teeth are extruded or missing, or discolored teeth are present in part of the arch, we are uncomfortable with what we see. Such an unbalanced dental composition is full of tension (Fig. 9, *bottom*).

Dominance

No discussion of visual ordering can ignore dominance. Notice how the biggest, brightest, and most centered objects attract our attention first. They are like a crescendo in music or a spotlight on a stage. When we are satisfied with our view of this most dominant element of the painting, we move on through the work as planned by the artist. We find ourselves being swept along major and secondary visual channels with components of lesser size or brightness. Finally, we are drawn back to the format in a self-renewing movement.

By virtue of their central position and their color contrast with the rest of the face, teeth are naturally the dominant element of the face. Because of their forward position, size, and brightness, the maxillary central incisors play the dominant role within the dental composition. Frush and Fisher [1–6] stated that stronger dominating elements lead to a more vigorous dental composition, whereas weaker dominating elements lead to monotony. Visual ordering begins with our attention drawn to the smile, particularly the teeth. Visual channels follow the lateral aspect of the teeth, consider the negative space in the buccal corridor, and evaluate the framing effect the contrasting lips provide, before either returning to the dominant central incisors or moving to other parts of the face (Fig. 1). It is appropriate that such a dominant element of the face receive considerable attention, as evidenced by the psychologic studies noted in the introduction of this discussion.

Economy

To bring out specific content or meaning, artists emphasize certain elements at the expense of others. This distortion helps to bring order and eliminate elements that distract or are unnecessarily complex (Fig. 11). Such economy is useful in our dental compositions, too, so that we may avoid distractive or confusing content (Fig. 4). Lacking check lines, stains, or color depth, bright white teeth may be associated with youth. Eliminating the display of clasps and metallic restorations is another way dentists use the principle of economy to avoid distraction and confusion. Such distrac-

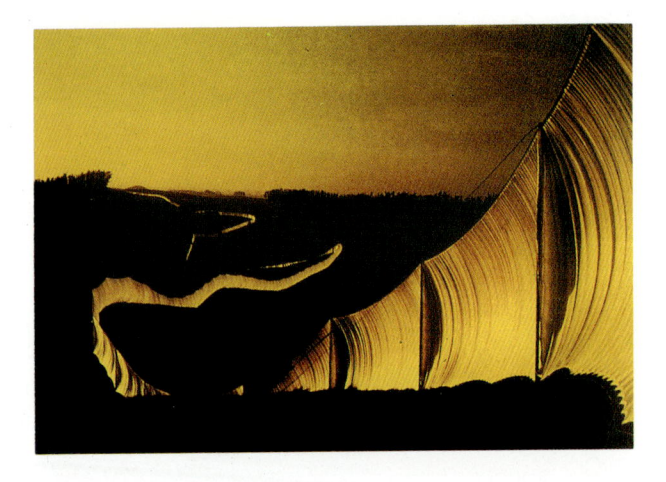

Fig. 8. In the "Running Fence," the eye is drawn from the forefront along an irregular line to the horizon, a simple example of visual forming. (Christo and Jean-Claude, "Running Fence, Sonoma and Marin Counties, California, 1972–76." *Copyright* 1976 by Christo, *photograph by* Jean-Claude; used with permission.)

tive elements would create visual channels that obscure the desired content of the smile composition, such as beauty, vitality, or masculinity.

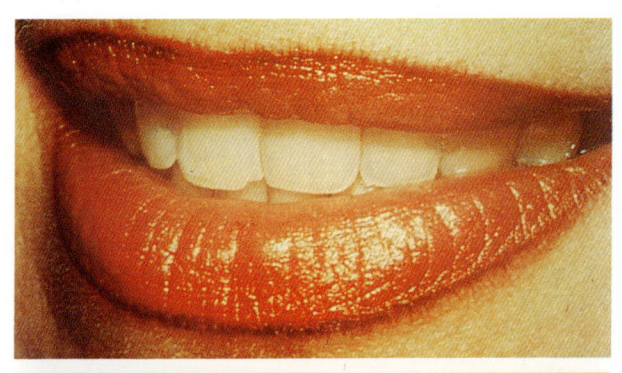

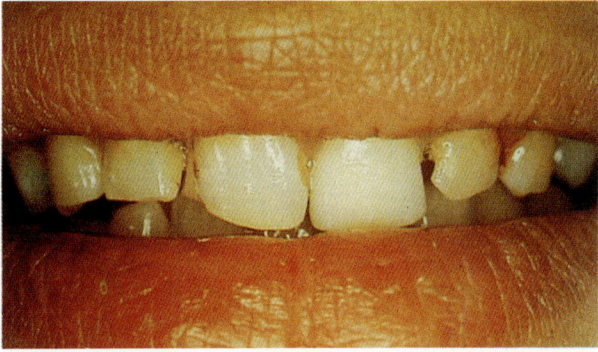

Fig. 9. All the elements of good art are present in this smile. (*From* Rufenacht [23••]; with permission.) **Bottom,** An unbalanced smile is full of tension.

Clinical application

I shall now review a practical case to demonstrate the application of the principles just discussed. Although the patient could have been evaluated solely according to dental esthetic rules, such as smile lines, the use of artistic concepts helped to provide a depth and feel for the meaning that resulted. These artistic concepts should be used in conjunction with—or even become a foundation for—the dental esthetic rules that already form a part of our training. Rufenacht [23••] wrote, "The appreciation of beauty, far from being related to the subjectivity of individual taste, requires methodic training for the promotion of individual feeling, in accordance with objective criteria."

An attractive 25-year-old woman complained that she was self-conscious about her smile (Fig. 12, *top*). Her front teeth were short, she said. Crowns had been placed on her front teeth by another dentist 4 years earlier. While speaking with her, I saw that her teeth distracted my gaze from her overall appearance, because the two central incisors were much brighter than the adjacent teeth, they were quite wide, and their gingival margins were a dark red. She had a very high smile line that showed as much gingiva as teeth. She worked at hiding her smile by covering her mouth with her hand or wetting her lips and then sealing them closed.

The discussion thus far describes our patient in typical dental terms. Consider this same patient, however, as an artist might. She is a young, attractive American. In our culture, we value a natural and ideally proportioned appearance. Because of the distraction of the bright wide crowns and gummy smile, our intuition immediately tells us something is wrong. We do not associate dental defects with young adults who attend to their appearance. Our eye might be more accepting of such defects in an older laborer. It turns out that the distortion created by unsightly crowns had now brought attention to a gummy smile that the patient has accepted for years. The crowns violate a sense of unity. The gummy smile violates the balance we expect.

In consultation with the patient, I used computer imaging to explore the effect various treatments might create. Our desire was to create a smile that would be seen as soft, beautiful, and in harmony with the rest of the face. Once we modified the primary distractive element of bright central incisors, their disproportionate size compared with the adjacent teeth became the new dominant distraction. When the widths of all four incisors were adjusted, the prominent gingiva and short teeth became the primary distractive element. Working out such details with sketches on the computer screen might been compared with the sketches Rembrandt used to develop his most effective presentation (Fig. 7). Other devices, such as wax-ups or composite mock-ups, may also be useful, but in all cases, we should expect to do our homework before beginning definitive treatment if want to achieve an artistic result.

The final result was accomplished by the kind of gingival resection described by Townsend [24•], replacing the existing crowns on the central incisors and making porcelain veneers for the lateral incisors. In the fi-

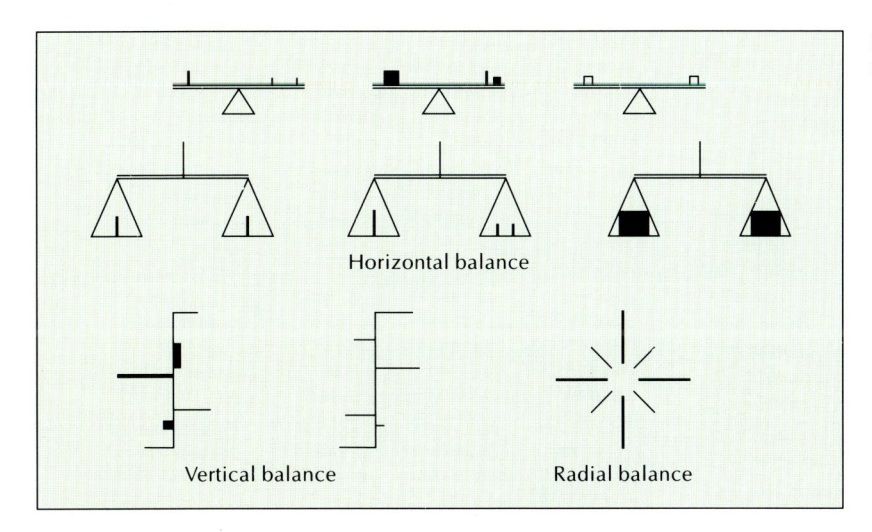

Fig. 10. Schematics of visual balance. (*Modified from* Ocvirk *et al.* [25••].)

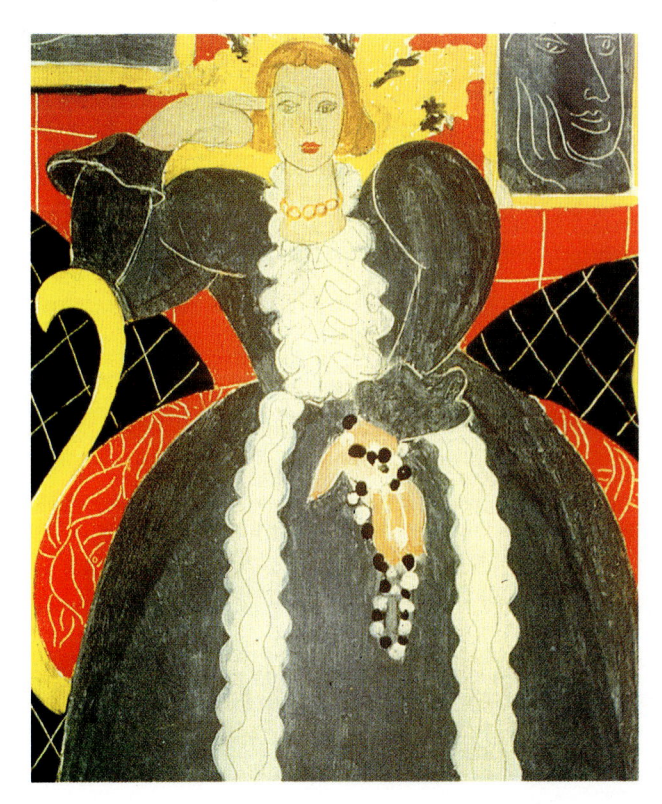

Fig. 11. In "Lady in Blue" (1937), Matisse began with a busy image and simplified it. (The Philadelphia Museum of Art, Philadelphia, PA; used with permission.)

sual channels. As our eye travels along these channels, we find subtle variations in tooth position, color, and shape that lend interest and personality to the composition. Numerous rounded lines help to create the desired softness, femininity, and youthful associations. If I were at liberty to show the entire face, we would see these concepts expanded beyond the borders of the lips.

nal result (Fig. 12, *bottom*) note that the vertical and horizontal proportion of the teeth are similar, but on different scales, in accordance with the golden proportion. The repetition of shapes develops harmony. The variation in size, which is also present in nature, creates interest. Similarly, the variation in color within each tooth and from tooth to tooth is interesting and attractive, and it provides separation between the tooth units. The smile lines created by the lips, incisal edges, and the gingival line are repeating lines that develop harmony. The dominant teeth, *ie*, the central incisors, attract our attention first, but not so much as to prevent it from moving laterally along the planned vi-

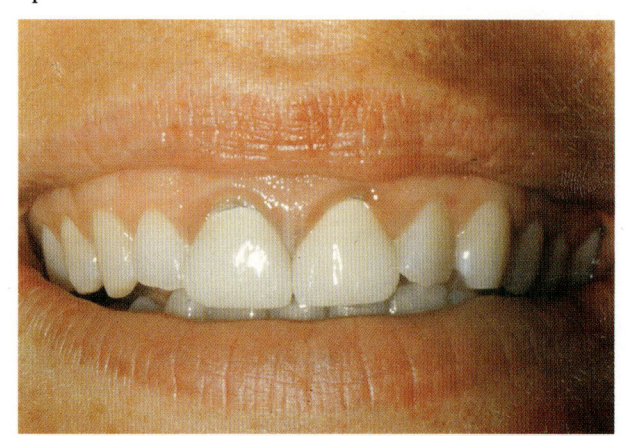

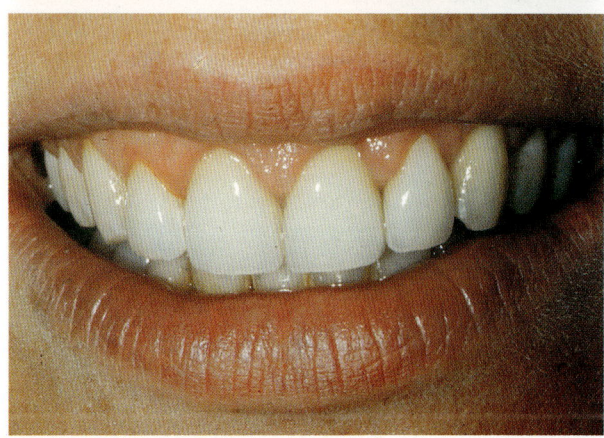

Fig. 12. Top, The distractive elements of this smile create tension. Intuitively, we know something is wrong. **Bottom,** After treatment, the smile is serene because harmony predominates. This soft, youthful, and feminine composition projects the content or meaning sought by the patient.

Conclusions

A study of the visual arts offers a fresh perspective on beauty in cosmetic dentistry. When we begin to use artistic skill in our smile compositions, the proportion and positional rules we have already learned for smile design become useful tools, rather than rigid masters. We are free to become artists as we serve the patrons of our art, our patients. This article has introduced the cosmetic dentist to principles of composition and discussed several personality traits of beauty. Those who wish to learn more about art and principles of composition might begin with a text such as *Art Fundamentals: Theory and Practice* [25••]. The integration of artistic principles and dental esthetic guidelines has been addressed by Rufenacht [23••]. Esthetics, the study of beauty in art and nature, comprises an entire school of thought in the fine arts. Public libraries and especially those associated with art museums offer other useful volumes on the subject.

References and recommended reading

Papers of particular interest, published within the annual period of review, have been highlighted as:
- • Of special interest
- •• Of outstanding interest.

1. Frush JP, Fisher RD: **Introduction to dentogenic restorations.** *J Prosthet Dent* 1955, 5:586–595.

2. Frush JP, Fisher RD: **How dentogenic restorations interpret the sex factor.** *J Prosthet Dent* 1956, 6:160–172.

3. Frush JP, Fisher RD: **How dentogenics interpret the personality factor.** *J Prosthet Dent* 1956, 6:441–449.

4. Frush JP, Fisher RD: **The age factor in dentogenics.** *J Prosthet Dent* 1957, 7:5–13.

5. Frush JP, Fisher RD: **The dynesthetic interpretation of the dentogenic concept.** *J Prosthet Dent* 1958, 8:558–581.

6. Frush JP, Fisher RD: **Dentogenics: its practical application.** *J Prosthet Dent* 1959, 9:914–921.

7. Kemnitzer DF: **Esthetics and the denture base.** *J Prosthet Dent* 1956, 4:603–615.

8. Pound E: **Esthetic dentures and their phonetic values.** *J Prosthet Dent* 1951, 1:98–111.

9. Macgregor F, Abel T, Lauer E, Weissman S: *Facial Deformities and Plastic Surgery: A Psychosocial Study.* New York: CC Thomas; 1953.

10. Goffman E: *Stigma: Notes on the Management of Spoiled Identity.* Englewood Cliffs: Prentice-Hall; 1963.

11. Crawford EC: **The face: an orthodontic perspective.** *Aust Orthod J* 1991, 12:13–22.

12. Lew KKK, Soh G, Loh E: **Ranking of facial profiles among Asians.** *J Esthetic Dent* 1992, 4:128–130.
    •

This study assesses facial profile preferences in an Asian population. By design, it recognizes ethnic and cultural influence on the perception of beauty. The study also refers to other studies of Asian and white populations' focus on the mouth as a primary determinant of facial attractiveness.

13. Terry RL: **Further evidence on components of facial attractiveness.** *Percept Mot Skills* 1977, 45:130–139.

14. Singer B: **Principles of esthetics.** *Curr Opin Cosmetic Dent* 1994, 2:6–12.

15. Singer B: **Fundamentals of esthetics.** In *Esthetic Dentistry:*
    • *A Clinical Approach to Techniques and Materials,* edn 1. Edited by Dale BG, Ascheim KW. Philadelphia: Lea & Febiger; 1993:5–13.

This text discusses color, light, and perception and how to manipulate them to create illusions in esthetic dentistry.

16. Farrow AL, Zarrinnia K, Azizi K: **Bimaxillary protrusion in black Americans: an esthetic evaluation and the treatment considerations.** *Am J Orthod Dentofacial Orthop* 1991, 104:240–250.

17. Phillips C, Tulloch C, Cann C IV: **Rating of facial attractiveness.** *Community Dent Oral Epidemiol* 1992, 20:214–220.

18. Czarnecki ST, Nanda RS, Currier GF: **Perceptions of a balanced facial profile.** *Am J Orthod Dentofacial Orthop* 1993, 104:180–187.

19. Rufenacht CR: **Introduction to esthetics.** In *Fundamentals of Esthetics,* edn 1. Chicago: Quintessence; 1990:11–31.

20. Morani AD: **Art in medical education, especially plastic**
    • **surgery.** *Aesthetic Plast Surg 1992,* 16:213–218.

This article encourages the incorporation of the study of art into the training of plastic surgeons for the purpose of developing a trained eye.

21. Newton E: *The Meaning of Beauty.* New York: McGraw-Hill; 1950.

22. Read H: *The Anatomy of Art: An Introduction to the Problems of Art and Aesthetics.* New York: Dodd, Mead, & Co.; 1932.

23. Rufenacht CR: *Fundamentals of Esthetics,* edn 1. Chicago:
    •• Quintessence Publishing Co.; 1990.

This is a dental text that integrates principles of art into esthetic guidelines well known to dentistry. It is a good source for further study, particularly if used in combination with texts on art and a study of esthetics.

24. Townsend CL: **Resective surgery: an esthetic application.**
    • *Quintessence Int* 1993, 24:523–542.

This article discusses the features of an "ideal" smile and several surgical modalities useful in modifying gingival architecture. The discussion covers important indications, potential risks of treatment, the use of stents to achieve predictable results, and suturing technique.

25. Ocvirk OC, Stinson RE, Wigg PR, Bone RO: *Art Fundamen-*
    •• *tals: Theory and Practice,* edn 6. Dubuque: Wm C Brown; 1990.

This undergraduate-level text for art students teaches principles of art composition. Much of the material in this article was taken from this text. This and subsequent editions are an excellent source for further study.

Thomas S. Valo, DDS, 6465 Monroe Street, Sylvania, OH 43560, USA.

Treating dental disharmony with mixed media

William M. Dorfman, DDS

Los Angeles, California, USA

The art of designing a new smile often involves more than one cosmetic dental procedure. It is not uncommon to combine media such as tooth whitening with porcelain veneers and crowns to create an entirely new smile. To maintain dental harmony, it is paramount that media are indistinguishable from each other and are consistent with the existing dentition.

One of the greatest challenges in dentistry is to blend cosmetic restorations with the color, form, and texture of an existing dentition. This challenge becomes increasingly difficult when different types of restorations and procedures are used adjacent to and in conjunction with each other to design a new smile.

Tooth whitening

In today's society, whiter, brighter teeth are considered a positive beauty enhancement. With the advent of take-home tooth whitening preparations and their proven safety and efficacy [1•,2,3•,4,5••,6,7], it is prudent to offer this service prior to attempting any cosmetic restorations. It is frustrating to spend many hours custom-staining porcelain crowns to a characterized Vita shade C3 dentition (Vita Zahnfabrik, Bad Saeckingen, FRG) and seating the perfectly matched restorations, and then to have the patient express a desire for a whiter smile at the 6-month recall. Had the whitening been completed first, shade selection would have been simplified because light tooth shades are easier to match than dark ones. Concurrently, the patient's esthetic demands would have been fulfilled.

There are two critical reasons why cosmetic restorations should not be color-selected and seated until at least 2 weeks after completion of the whitening procedure. First, the treated teeth will be at their whitest the 1st day after completion of the whitening process. Time is needed for the color to stabilize; only then can the new restorations be placed without the risk of an immediate color shift in the adjacent natural teeth. In the future, with newly fabricated trays, the patient will be able to perform "touch up" whitening for a few nights every 4 to 12 months to maintain the desired shade. Second, immediately after the use of a hydrogen peroxide–based whitening system, the shear bond strength of composite resin to enamel is reduced [8•,9]. However, a 2-week waiting period appears to be sufficient to eliminate the significant difference in bond strength of composite resin to enamel and dentin [9,10] (Fig. 1).

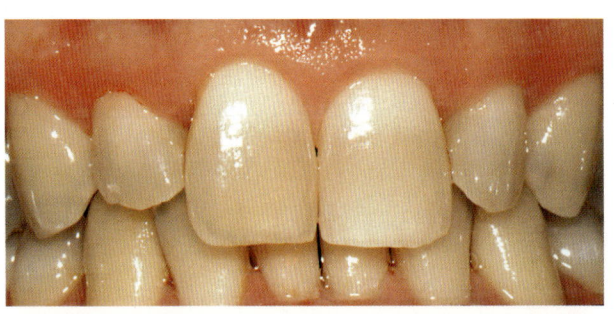

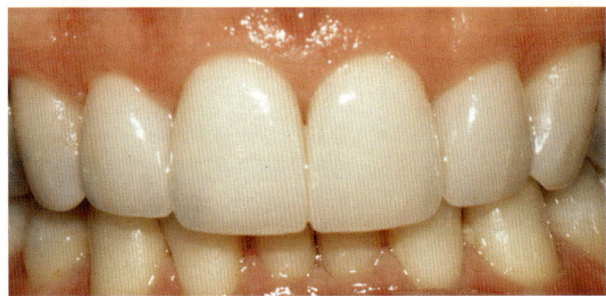

Fig. 1. Top, Before treatment. **Bottom**, One year after bleaching, gingival recontouring of tooth 9, attachment of porcelain veneers to teeth 7 to 10, and application of mesial incisal composites to teeth 6 and 11.

Matching porcelain veneers

One of the greatest benefits of porcelain veneers is the lifelike appearance attained by the translucency of the porcelain. However, this benefit becomes a hindrance when one or more of the teeth involved in the restorative procedure are severely discolored (Fig. 2, *top*).

Three factors determine the final shade of a porcelain veneer: 1) the color and opacity of the porcelain; 2) the color and opacity of the luting resin; and 3) the underlying color of the enamel or dentin. Altering any one of these factors will influence the final shade of the restoration.

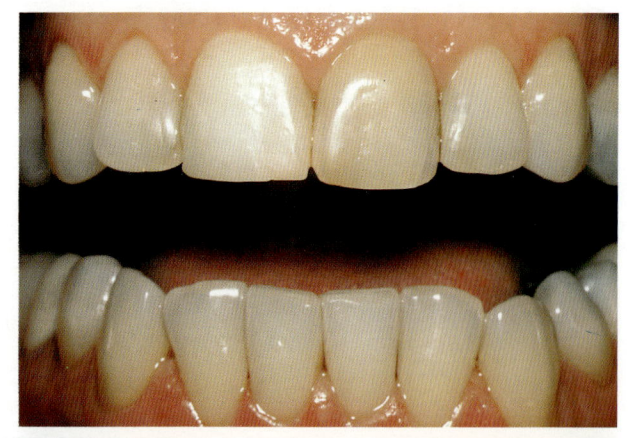

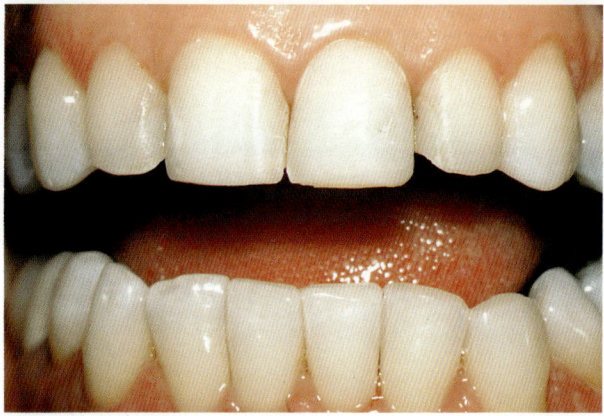

Fig. 2. Top, Tooth 8 is a discolored, endodontically treated tooth. **Bottom,** The shade of tooth 8 is altered with a microfill or hybrid composite to match the prepared shade of tooth 9.

Some problems may occur if color correction of a single discolored tooth is attempted in the porcelain or luting agent:

The color correction may over- or undercompensate for the problem, because there is no exact formula available to predict results.

The opacity used to block out the undesired color may alter the optical properties of the restoration and prevent a perfect blend with adjacent teeth.

Luting resin cements, which are viscous enough to allow seating of the veneers, will also alter the final shade depending on the space between the tooth and the porcelain veneer. Unfortunately, it is difficult to determine the thickness of the luting resin when seating veneers. There is also the problem of controlling the amount of shade-modifying tint that remains in a veneer as it is being seated and the excess is extruded.

The most predictable way to acquire a perfect shade match is to make the color correction on the prepared tooth (Fig. 2, *bottom*) with a microfill or hybrid composite. Bond strength of composite resin luting cements to microfill and hybrid composite on the tooth is excellent, provided the microfill has been placed recently and prepared and sandblasted just prior to cementation [11]. The end result is that the final restoration will appear exactly the same on the discolored tooth, because it will exhibit the same optical properties as the adjacent teeth (Fig. 3).

Matching porcelain veneers and crowns

As illustrated above, the most predictable way to establish a perfect color match on different restorations is to use identical materials with identical optical properties. When the matching of translucent porcelain veneers to adjacent porcelain-fused-to-metal crowns is attempted, an obvious esthetic problem is the grayness that remains from the metal in the crowns and a lack of through-and-through translucency. It is therefore advantageous to use an all-porcelain crown instead of a procelain-fused-to-metal crown. Some of the new all-porcelain crowns available, such as IPS Empress Crown (Ivoclar North America, Amherst NY), exhibit as much as 90% more resistance to fracture than conventional all-porcelain crowns when loaded axially and obliquely [12].

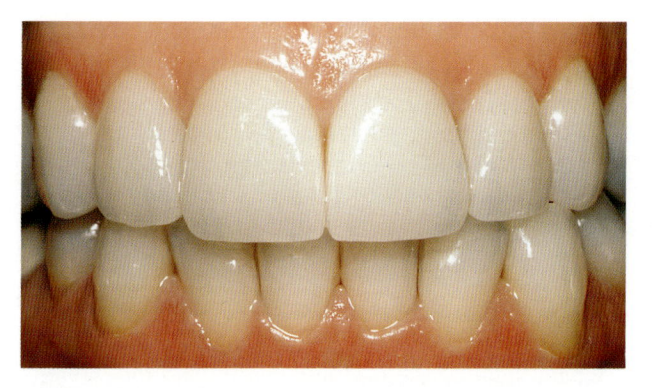

Fig. 3. The final restorations for this patient consist of porcelain veneers on teeth 6 to 11, all of which exhibit identical optical properties.

Once the core of the crown is divested, it can be cut back. To produce identical coloration, lower fusing veneer porcelain may then be layered on the core in exactly the same manner as it is on the die of the adjacent veneer teeth (Fig. 4).

Conclusions

When whitening teeth, always wait a sufficient amount of time prior to placing cosmetic dental restorations [13•]. The most predictable way to correct dental shade disharmony with mixed media is to make color corrections on the prepared tooth. Once the shade correction has been established, the restorations can be fabricated in the standard fashion. For mixed media cases involving crowns and veneers, it is beneficial to duplicate the

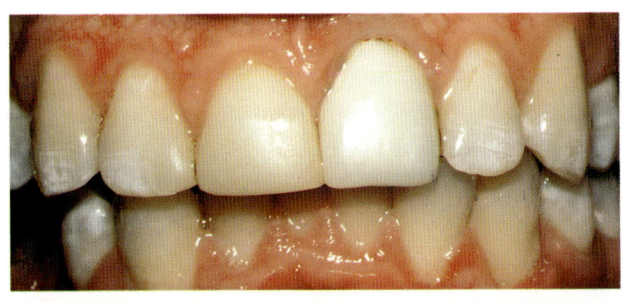

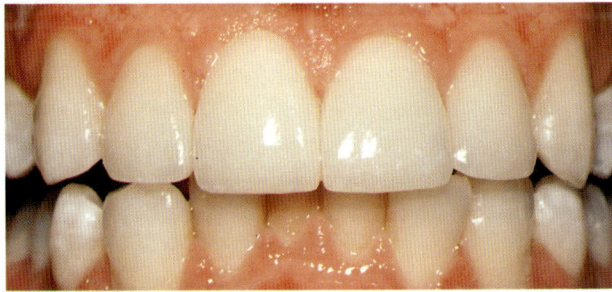

Fig. 4. Top, Before treatment. Note the discolored composite on tooth 8 and the failing crown on tooth 9. **Bottom,** Immediately after application of take-home tooth whitening, attachment of porcelain veneers on teeth 7, 8, and 10, and mounting of an IPS Empress Crown (Ivoclar North America, Amherst, NY) on tooth 9.

optical properties of the veneered tooth in the crown. This may be accomplished by matching the crown core to the desired shade and then layering simultaneously the same porcelain on the veneers and the crown.

References and recommended reading

Papers of particular interest, published within the annual period of review, have been highlighted as:
- Of special interest
- •• Of outstanding interest

1. Reinhardt JW, Eivins SE, Swift EJ Jr, Denehy GE: **A clinical
• study of nightguard vital bleaching.** *Quintessence Int* 1993, 24:379–384.
Indicates that bleaching treatment is effective in most cases and causes no tissue inflammation or significant tooth sensitivity.

2. Haywood VB: **The Food and Drug Administration and its influence on home bleaching.** *Curr Opin Cosmetic Dent* 1993, 1:12–18.

3. Gegauff AG, Rosenstiel SF, Langhout KJ, Johnston WM: **Eval-
• uating tooth color change from carbamide peroxide gel.** *J Am Dent Assoc* 1993, 124:65–72.
After carbamide tooth bleaching, no permanent changes were found in either pulpal or gingival health.

4. Nakamura T, Nakajima H, Salimee P, Hino T, Maruyama T: **Effect of bleaching on vital discoloured teeth: a colorimetric evaluation in three patients.** *Asian J Aesthet Dent* 1993, 1:25–28.

5. Haywood VB: **Considerations and variations of dentist-
•• prescribed, home-applied vital tooth-bleaching techniques.** *Compendium* 1994, Suppl 17:S616–S621.
Suggests that dentist-supervised take-home bleaching has the lowest risk level and is 96% successful.

6. Simon JF, Allen H, Woodson RG, Eilers AS: **Efficacy of vital home bleaching** *J Calif Dent Assoc* 1993, 21:72–75.

7. Goldstein GR, Kiremidjian-Schumacher L: **Bleaching: is it safe and effective?** *J Prosthet Dent* 1993, 69:325–328.

8. Garcia-Godoy F, Dodge WW, Donohue M, O'Quinn JA:
• **Composite resin bond strength after enamel bleaching.** *Oper Dent* 1993, 18:144–147.
This study reveals that the shear bond strength of composite resin is significantly reduced for 24 hours after enamel bleaching.

9. Titley KC, Torneck CD, Ruse ND, Krmec D: **Adhesion of a resin composite to bleached and unbleached human enamel.** *J Endod* 1993, 19:112–115.

10. Cullen DR, Nelson JA, Sandrik JL: **Peroxide bleaches: effect on tensile strength of composite resins.** *J Prosthet Dent* 1993, 69:247–249.

11. Nixon R: **Masking severely tetracycline stained teeth with porcelain veneers.** *Pract Periodontics Aesthet Dent* 1990, 2:14–18.

12. Ludwig, K: **Studies on the ultimate strength of all-ceramic crowns.** *Dent Lab* 1991, 5:647–651.

13. Weinstein AR: **Esthetic applications of restorative materials
• and techniques in the anterior dentition.** *Dent Clin North Am* 1993, 37:391–409.
Suggests that that most conservative noninvasive techniques for cosmetic dentistry should be tried first, and that often, bleaching and direct (*ie*, partial) bonding are all that is needed.

William M. Dorfman, DDS, 2080 Century Park East, Suite 1101, Los Angeles, CA 90067, USA.

Color management of cosmetic restorations

Kenneth L. Glick, DDS

Don Mills, Ontario, Canada

Ideally, a cosmetic restoration should be indistinguishable from the surrounding unrestored dentition. The cosmetic dentist faces the challenging task of creating the restoration using materials that do not possess the light-transmitting properties of natural tooth structures. A thorough knowledge of the physical and physiologic properties of light, color production and perception, and skill in the art of color matching can lead to rewarding success.

The increasing role of cosmetic procedures in modern dental practice has brought with it increased demands on the dental practitioner. Patients are becoming more sophisticated and are less accepting of inferior results. Nothing is more obvious and immediately noticeable than even a slight shade discrepancy between the natural dentition and the media used to restore it, whether it be porcelain, resin, or any variation thereof. As a consequence, the practitioner must be well-educated in the theory, science, and art of color management. This knowledge will serve well in communicating with technical support staff and in achieving highly acceptable esthetic results.

It is unfortunate that despite the critical role that color management plays in the success of an esthetic restoration, institutional instruction in this subject on an undergraduate level remains sketchy at best [1]. Moreover, the best reference has been out of print for several years [2]. Searching the recent literature yields only a few references to color management, because most authors assume that the reader is fully knowledgeable and skilled in this everyday aspect of dental practice.

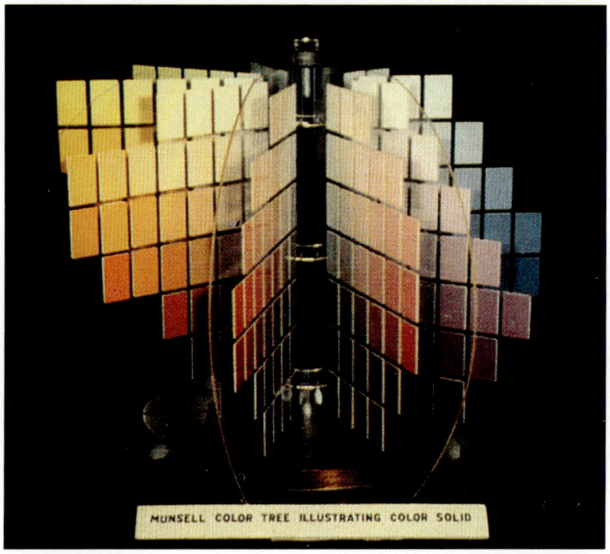

Fig. 1. The Munsell color system arranges color logically. Each arm represents one hue. Chroma increases as one moves from the center to the periphery, and value increases from bottom to top. Unfortunately, no such system exists for dentistry.

Color science

As Monetti [3] stated: "Failures to select acceptable shades often can be traced to lack of understanding of basic color science."

In discussing the scientific basis of color theory, Glick [4••] wrote, "It is necessary to define and understand the terms by which we interpret and describe the quality and quantity of the colors we discuss" so that we all "speak the same language."

Hue is the name of the wavelength of light we commonly call a color. *Chroma* refers to the amount, or saturation, of the color present. *Value* represents the relative lightness or darkness of a color (Fig. 1).

Glick [5••] also reviewed the three methods by which color is mixed (additive, subtractive, and partitive) and described the problem of metamerism in terms of the physical property of spectral reflectance that produces it. After a review of the physical factors involved in the phenomenon of color, Glick considered the physiologic factors involved in color vision. Factors inherent in the structure and function of the human eye influence our ability to see color and can be used to our benefit if they are understood. For instance, because we know that the rods of the eye can judge for value only and that they are peripheral to the more centrally located cones, we recommend that an operator should squint when judging the value of a shade selection. Squinting brings the rods into greater play and thus enhances the ability to compare values.

The phenomenon of color blindness was also discussed. Because approximately 9% of men exhibit some form of color vision defect, testing for this defect can determine if it is a factor in color decision-making for the individual practitioner. Color blindness could lead to the decision, by some practitioners, to have a female auxiliary staff member select the shades.

Another factor that affects the ability to select shades and that is often overlooked is age. As the eye ages, the lens and the cornea "become less efficient in transmitting light and they may yellow" [5••]. This factor alone may lead to incorrect shade selection as the practitioner gets older, and it should be taken into consideration.

Finally, the effect of hue adaptation should be understood and compensated for. The depletion of photopigments in the eye reduces the operator's ability to distinguish between the color of a shade guide tab and that of the tooth being matched. By considering this factor, the operator can alter shade selection technique to minimize this effect.

Shade-matching environment

A proper environment increases the likelihood of successful shade matching [3,6••]. The quality of the light source under which shade selection occurs is most important. It should produce "a color temperature of 5500°K, a spectral curve like that of standard daylight, and a color rendition index of 90" [3]. I recommend the use of color-corrected, so-called *daylight* fluorescent tubes if they satisfy the previous criteria.

Although the quality of light is important, the quantity of light is a factor that is often overlooked. The recommended minimum in each operatory is 150 foot-candles, or the equivalent of 12 120-cm, color-corrected fluorescent tubes in an operatory with 240-cm ceilings and 9 m² of floor space.

Both Monetti [3] and Glick [6••] agreed that once adequate quality and quantity of light have been provided, the environment in which shades will be viewed must be considered. Reflecting surfaces in the operatory should be of high value with white ceilings and neutral gray or pastel blue walls, cabinets, and counters. "Heavy colors such as green, blue and red may influence selection" [3]. The practitioner should also consider other surfaces that can be controlled, such as bibs and uniforms, and those over which there is little control, such as patient clothing. All these elements will affect the success of the shade-matching process.

Selection technique

Based on our knowledge of the physical characteristics and physiologic factors involved in color production and interpretation, and provided a proper environment has been established, a standardized, routine technique for shade selection can be established. This will simplify the task of proper shade selection (Fig. 2).

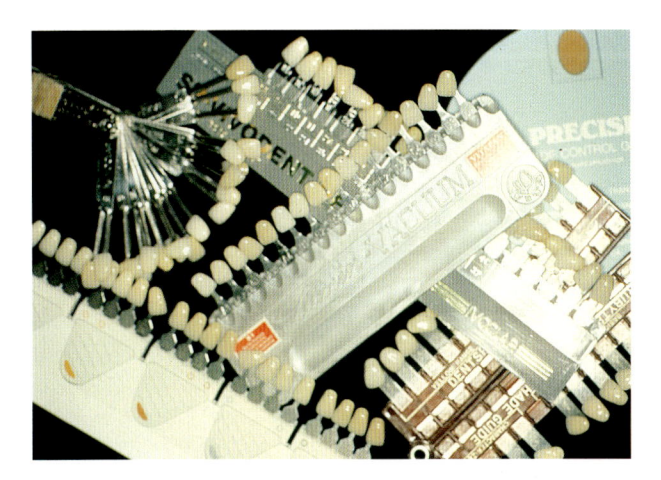

Fig. 2. Shade guides are used to select the proper color of restorations. A wide variety of guides from which to choose should be available.

Glick's [6••] 12 steps comprise a standardized shade-matching procedure:

1. Clean the tooth to be matched

2. Check for apparent value and dominant hue and select the likeliest shade guide tab (Fig. 3)

3. Moisten the selected shade guide tab

4. Hold the selected shade guide tab next to the tooth being matched

5. Squint to appraise for value

6. Note hue differences and chroma levels

7. Limit viewing to 5 seconds at a time; stare at a blue card to counteract the effects of hue adaptation, thereby restoring visual color acuity

8. View with lips both relaxed and reflected; consider the color of the gingiva when determining the shade; gingival color varies: it may be red, pink or orange; the restored tooth color should blend harmoniously with the gingival and lip colors [7•]

9. Use multiple, *ie*, different, light sources

10. Select a shade of higher value and lower chroma if no ideal match is available; it is easier to lower value and raise chroma if the restoration's shade must be modified

11. Modify the guide (first breaking the glaze with a sandblaster such as the Microetcher [Danville Engineering, Danville, CA]) with metal oxide colorants such as GC Orbit (G. C. America, Chicago, IL)

12. Submit the shade tab to the laboratory along with a full and complete prescription

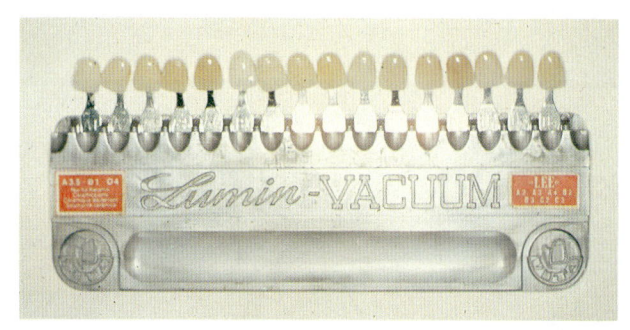

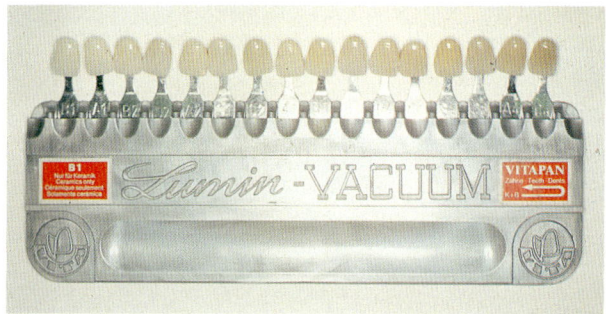

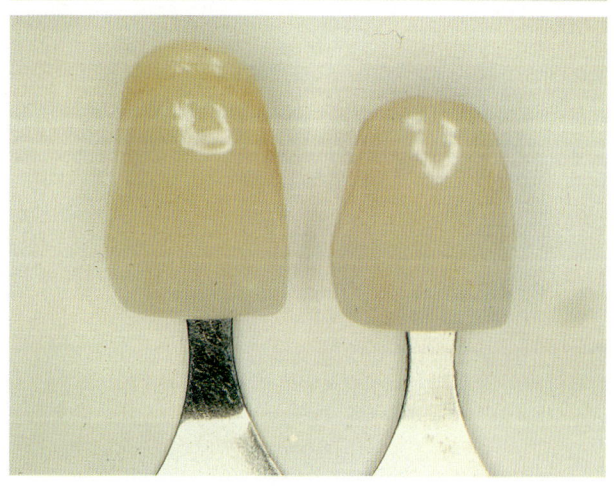

Fig. 3. Shade guides may be arranged by hue family (*top panel*) or by value (*center panel*). Removing the neck of a shade guide (*bottom panel*) eliminates the color distortion caused by characterization of the neck shade.

Miller *et al.* [7•] stated, "After shade selection, effectively communicating the desired information to the laboratory technician may still present a major problem." They recommended the use of two diagrams when there is variation from the standard color in the manufacturer's shade guides (Fig. 4). "A facial view is used to indicate the position of the various shades, while a proximal view will tell the technician how the body and enamel porcelains should be layered," they advised [7•]. For effective communication between the practitioner and the laboratory, as much supplementary material as is needed should be supplied [6••]. This may include all or some of diagrams, models, photographs, shade tabs, custom shade tabs, and luster tabs. Williamson [8] described a technique for custom shade guide fabrication. Glick [6••] indicated that form, surface texture, and glaze affected the overall success of the color-matching process, and that these are more important to the overall success of a case than color itself.

Controlling form and contour is necessary for both esthetics and periodontal health. This factor dictates that porcelain should not be overcontoured, and it does require some bulk in which to develop color. Strict attention must be paid to ensure that adequate tooth reduction takes place. Ideally, there should be enough space for a minimum of 1 mm cervically with 1.5 mm midlabially and a 2.5-mm reduction of the incisal edge [6••].

It is a curious fact that dental school instruction creates pulp-shy operators. Although protection of the pulp is a major concern, it leads to the frequently seen problem of high-value porcelain-bonded-to-metal crowns resulting from conservative underpreparation.

The underpreparation of teeth places the technician between the proverbial rock and a hard place. If the crown is constructed according to the esthetic requirements of three layers of restorative materials (metal, opaque porcelain, and body porcelain), the resulting crown will be overbuilt, and periodontal ramifications will result. On the other hand, if the demands of form and function are given greater precedence than those of esthetics, then a high-value crown will result because the technician must sacrifice thickness of the semitranslucent body porcelain, allowing the high-value opaque layer to dominate.

Although crown form is a critical factor, as Glick [6••] stated, "A tooth that is acceptable in form or color may still not blend with its neighbors if its surface texture is incorrect."

Surface texture is the major contributor to the manner in which light reflects from the labial surface of a tooth to the eye viewing it. It is recommended that surface texture be placed by the dentist at a try-in appointment. This is preferable to having the technician texturize the surface because the model with which the technician is working may not contain an accurate record of fine surface detail.

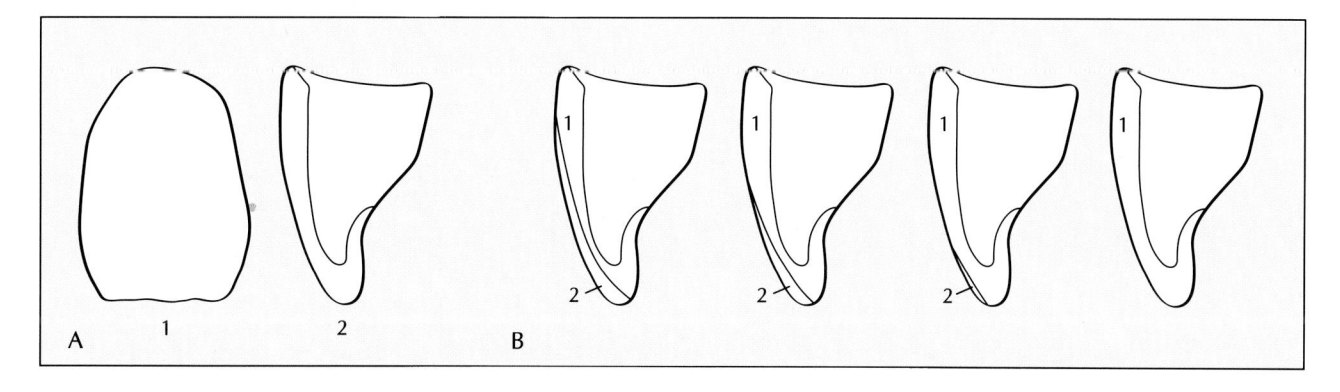

Fig. 4. A, Facial (*1*) and proximal (*2*) view diagrams are used to illustrate both the position of various shades and the layering of body and enamel porcelains for the technician. **B,** Proximal diagrams illustrating various arrangements of body (*1*) and incisal (*2*) porcelains. (*Modified from* Miller *et al.* [7•].)

The final influence on ultimate success or failure in color management is control of the surface luster, or glaze, of the finished restoration. Williamson and Breeding [9•] described the effect of surface luster on the appearance of ceramic restorations and discussed a technique for making a luster tab similar to a shade tab.

According to Williamson and Breeding and to Glick [6••], the quality of the final glaze influences the perception of chroma, value, and translucency. Highly glazed surfaces reflect more light, so that they appear to be higher in value, lower in chroma, and less translucent, whereas low surface glaze produces lower value, higher chroma, and more translucency. It is therefore important to communicate to the technician the degree of surface luster required to achieve a successful restoration.

Special situations

More and more frequently, cosmetic dental solutions are being demanded for difficult esthetic problems. In particular, treatment of teeth discolored by tetracycline-based medications creates difficulty for the cosmetic dentist.

Using basic color theory, Yamada [10•] described a technique for using complementarily colored porcelain in the construction of porcelain veneers, which was designed to neutralize the underlying tooth shade to "produce a grayish tone to which a white modifier is added to increase the value of the color." Yamada's article provides a useful illustration of a novel application of basic color theory to a difficult yet common esthetic dilemma. The conventional solution, using an opaque masking porcelain, often leads to overly white, unnatural-looking teeth.

Conclusions

Color management in cosmetic dentistry is an art based on science. To produce excellent results, the cosmetic practitioner must be well-versed in color management theory and technique. In the future, research such as that done by Ishikawa-Nagai *et al.* [11,12] may lead to excellent color management by coupling a spectrophotometer with a computer. Until that day, however, we must rely on the skill and knowledge of the trained dental professional.

References and recommended reading

Papers of particular interest, published within the annual period of review, have been highlighted as:
- • Of special interest
- •• Of outstanding interest.

1. Goodkind RJ, Loupe MJ: **Teaching of color in predoctoral dental education in 1988.** *J Prosthet Dent* 1992, 67:713–717.

2. Preston J, Bergen SF: *Color Science and Dental Art*. St. Louis: CV Mosby; 1980.

3. Monetti L: **Ceramic shade selection: by whom, where and under what circumstances.** *Trends Tech Contemp Dent Lab* 1993, 10:96–99.

4. Glick K: **Color and shade selection in cosmetic dentistry.** *J Am Acad Cosmetic Dent* December 1993: 7–10.
•• This article discusses the language used in describing color to establish a common reference vocabulary. The physical properties of light and the ways it combines to produce color phenomena are discussed.

5. Glick K: **Color and shade selection in cosmetic dentistry: part II.** *J Am Acad Cosmetic Dent* March 1994: 9–11.
•• This article describes the physiology of sight and color vision, with emphasis on its impact on shade selection.

6. Glick K: **Color and shade selection in cosmetic dentistry: part III.** *J Am Acad Cosmetic Dent* Summer 1994: 15–20.
•• This article discusses the establishment of a proper in-office shade selection environment and a standard technique for ensuring correct

shade selection. Other factors that affect the final overall appearance of restorations are described.

7. Miller A, Long J, Cole J, Staffanou R: **Shade selection and laboratory communication.** *Quintessence Int* 1993, 24:305–309.
• A discussion of the importance of and methods for communicating shades to the dental laboratory.

8. Williamson RT: **Methods for aesthetic evaluation in replacement of ceramic fixed prosthetics.** *Pract Periodontics Aesthet Dent* 1993, 5:47–54.

9. Williamson RT, Breeding LC: **Make luster tabs for use in matching texture of porcelain surfaces.** *J Prosthet Dent* 1993, 69:536–537.
• Describes a simple technique for fabricating luster tabs for use during shade selection procedures.

10. Yamada K: **Porcelain laminate veneers for discolored teeth using complementary colors.** *Int J Prosthodont* 1993, 6:242–247.
• This article presents a unique approach to masking tetracycline-stained teeth using basic knowledge of the principles of color mixing.

11. Ishikawa-Nagai S, Sawafuji F, Tsuchitoi H, Sato RR, Ishibashi K: **Using a computer color-matching system in color reproduction of porcelain restorations: part 2. Color reproduction of stratiform layered porcelain samples.** *Int J Prosthodont* 1993, 6:522–527.

12. Ishikawa-Nagai S, Sato RR, Shiraishi A, Ishibashi K: **Using a computer color-matching system in color reproduction of porcelain restorations: part 3. A newly developed spectrophotometer designed for clinical application.** *Int J Prosthodont* 1994 7:50–55.

Kenneth L. Glick, DDS, 10 Wynford Heights Crescent, Suite 140, Don Mills, Ontario, Canada M3C 1K8.

Restoring the aging dentition

Jacqueline Dzierzak, DMD

Chicago, Illinois, USA

The aging of the population has put new demands on the range and capabilities of the dentist. Patients are no longer satisfied with the straightforward restoration of their mouths. They are demanding a more youthful appearance as an essential element of therapy. To provide this element, the dentist must have a thorough understanding of the physiology of tooth and facial aging, the treatments available, and the problems and limitations that might be incurred.

Aging is an inevitable fact of life. From the time we are conceived, our genes lead our body through a series of changes ranging from growth and development to maturation, aging, and deterioration. This process appears to be not only programmed genetically but also influenced by our lifestyle and environment. Whereas past generations had little recourse but to lament their passing youth, our aging population is aggressively looking for and finding ways to retain younger, healthier bodies longer than ever before.

Through science and research, we are better able to understand the mechanism of change and apparently alter the aging process. In the past, it was considered a fact of life that once persons reached adulthood, they would lose their teeth and wear dentures for the remainder of their lives. At one time, dentists even recommended the extraction of the teeth early on to prevent pyorrhea. With an understanding of the periodontal disease process, a significant portion of the population are retaining their natural dentition throughout adulthood. Today, moreover, the adult market has split into a medically compromised segment and a relatively healthy segment. Not only is the new adult population healthier and more dentally aware than any preceding generation, but they want to retain their teeth, their ability to chew, smile, eat and function, and their youthful appearance.

Clinical techniques have previously been determined by restorative materials and methods that could restore lost or missing tooth structure but were fairly limited in their overall esthetic results. Techniques such as supragingival preparations and margins, the use of amalgam restorative materials and gold occlusal restorations may have been acceptable in the past, but they are no longer accepted by the visually concerned adult consumer of today. Dentistry is in the process of a transition from disease eradication to a kind of holistic medicine, in which health, beauty, and function are inseparable.

Today's dentistry must now focus not only on the replacement and restoration of tooth structure, but also on understanding the effect of material and treatment selection on image enhancement for the creation of a beautiful smile. Old artificial restorative materials such as amalgam and gold made the teeth look dark, dirty, defective, and unnatural. The new cosmetic materials create a white, bright, sexy, natural-appearing dentition, resulting in a smile that appears to have never been affected by disease. This smile looks normal and natural, a simulation and recreation of the real thing.

Today's society is also asking dentistry to produce a smile that looks 10 to 15 years younger than the patient's chronologic age. We are redefining what aging is all about. It is about the retention of youth as opposed to "graceful aging," getting old, or being called *geriatric*. In looking at dentistry from this new perspective, one must understand the physiology of aging and the effects that aging has on the facial architecture, the dental and periodontal support, and the functional interrelationship of these structures. Once these things are understood, the patient and the dentist can construct a treatment plan that will not only replace the missing structures but also confer a more pleasing and youthful appearance to the face and the smile.

The physiology of tooth aging

The aging of a tooth takes place from the time a tooth erupts into the oral cavity. At that time, the enamel is as thick as it will ever be and most likely as brilliant as it will ever be. As the tooth is subjected to mouth acids, foods, and the abrasive effects of toothbrush and toothpaste, there is a progressive microscopic alteration of the surface and the dimension of the enamel: it begins to wear down. Concurrently, the pulp and dentin undergo a transformation. They are subjected to heat, cold, pressures, trauma, and almost constant stimulation. With each of these insults, the pulp responds by stimulation and formation of secondary dentin. The pulp becomes smaller, while the dentin becomes thicker. As the nutrients and vascularity in the dentin decrease, the dentin begins to sclerose and increase in hardness. This process, combined with the decrease in the enamel layer, causes the tooth to appear darker. No matter how hard the patient brushes, the tooth will never regain its original color. Other changes that occur simultaneously include thermal cracking of the enamel: wear of the incisal, lingual, and occlusal surfaces with increased stain uptake; and alteration of position, contour, texture and occlusal relationships, to name a few. In cases of tetracycline staining, a progressive darkening of the photoactivated chemical within the tooth may also be noted. Alone, these changes cause a significant degree of shade shifting over the years. Combined with cleaning and dietary habits, they may accelerate the process.

While the tooth is losing its vitality or whiteness, other mechanisms of action are also coming into play. A person's hygiene habits dictate the amount of stain and debris accumulating supra- and subgingivally. These accumulations affect the color, vitality, and luster of the enamel. Traditional tooth cleaning, scaling, and root planing procedures may improve the color of the teeth, particularly if periodontal disease is brought under control and tissue color returns to normal. However, this method of removing debris has relatively little effect on the type of discoloration caused by food absorption staining. Food and beverage stains will frequently penetrate into the interstitial spaces of the enamel. Once penetration occurs, it is impossible for the patient to remove the discolorations routinely. This type of staining is also progressive in nature.

Treatment

Treatment may include plaque removal (as opposed to just brushing, flossing, and rubber tipping), which is the key to the successful treatment and maintenance of the adult patient's tooth and tissue color. Those patients who grew up scrub-brushing their teeth usually experienced alterations in the position of the tissue and a resultant increase in root sensitivity. These patients are reluctant to have their teeth cleaned owing to the hypersensitivity they experience with the use of ultrasonic cleaners, prophyjets, polishing agents, and cold-water sprays. The introduction of ultrasoft toothbrushes and rotary plaque removal instruments and the use of medicating and desensitizing agents such as neutral sodium fluoride have done wonders in reducing the pain that patients experience.

Additional augmentive procedures, such as connective tissue grafting, can prevent tissues from further recession and in some cases may be used to obtain root coverage. This is a welcome relief for those who have endured root sensitivity for prolonged periods of time. Similar augmentation procedures can be used to re-create a normal contour for a receding ridge so that the emergence contour of a pontic appears similar to that of the adjacent natural teeth.

New materials such as Goretex (Gore & Associates, Putzbrunn, FRG) and root-form multiple- and single-tooth implants are giving hope to those patients whose teeth in the past may have been destined for extraction. Techniques using periodontal plastic and other esthetic procedures are designed to enhance the final result by limiting or eliminating visual distractions such as variation in tooth length, inconsistency in gingival tissue margins, variability of emergence contours, and shadowing or absence of all or parts of the papillae, all of which mar the appearance of the smile.

Periodontists and general dentists together are planning cases that preserve the esthetic integrity of the dental arch, rather than restricting treatment to resection procedures designed solely for disease eradication. This quantum leap has resulted in improved esthetic results with fewer restorative complications and higher level of satisfaction among patients.

With the aging of the population, the design of treatment plans must take into account several factors:

- Any medical, local or systemic changes to the patient's health

- The use of medications that may affect surgical treatment or postoperative healing

- Changes in the vascularity of the tissues

- The patient's ability to maintain long-term periodontal support

- Bone changes such as osteoporosis

- Changes in nutrition

Not only do these changes affect fully dentulous adults, but they must be monitored in partially and fully edentulous patients.

Facial alterations with aging

Several different mechanisms cause alterations in facial contours and subsequently affect the age of the smile. I shall briefly present a few significant factors here, but readers should refer to a competent plastic surgery text for a more comprehensive discussion.

As the face ages, the tissues lose elasticity. The upper lip contour increases, and the incisal edge decreases. The process is exacerbated and accelerated by the bodily effects of gravitational droop. Cheeks sag, jowls appear, and the face takes on an older, more tired appearance. The skin color and vascularity pale with increasing age, while tooth color darkens, making the teeth look shorter, more recessive, and older. Facial and muscular support is altered owing to the wear that takes place on the facial, incisal, and occlusal surfaces of the teeth (Fig. 1).

Orthodontists have long known and written about the physiologic movement of the teeth in the mandibular arch that results in a decrease in the intercanine distance. This constriction of the dental arch can create crowding, a change in the interproximal contact relationships, alterations in centric occlusal stops and protrusive guidance, wear or the accelerated movement of certain teeth and the disuse and supraeruption of others. The lower arch may show signs of variable height and position rather than the straight look that it may once have had. It also presents problems of maintenance, owing to tighter interproximal contacts, alterations in bony and soft tissue contours, and increasing patterns of stain, plaque, and tartar accumulation.

Treating early crowding of the lower anterior arch with enamel reshaping or orthodontic repositioning can stabilize the dentition for a lifetime. More severe crowd-

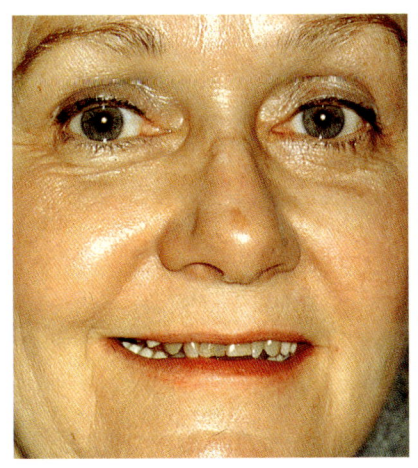

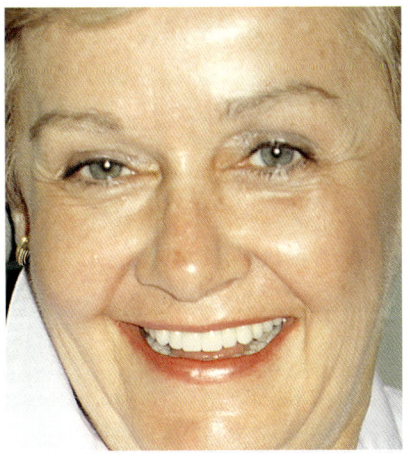

Fig. 1. Left, A woman in her mid-60s noticed progressive alterations in the color, length and position of her teeth through the years, which made her face appear older than it was. **Right,** After therapy, the face and smile were interrelated. The patient felt and looked relaxed and confident.

ing may necessitate strategic single tooth extraction followed by orthodontic closure of the residual spaces.

Incisal and occlusal wear, whether physiologic or pathologic, is reflected in changes of tooth form and length. Teeth that once displayed varying degrees of incisal length and incisal edge show and followed the smile line contour of the lower lip tend to flatten on the incisal edge. Incisal embrasure spaces, which created a youthful appearance, decrease in dimension and assume a straighter incisal appearance. Incisal edges that were once thin and translucent begin to appear thick and flat with loss of the incisal enamel and decreased translucency.

The wear patterns of the maxillary teeth also show thinning of the lingual incisal contour and produce the enamel chipping and shearing pattern that is common among older patients. The mandibular teeth show loss of incisal facial enamel and increasing amounts of dentin exposure and discoloration over time. Procedures such as enamel recontouring enhance the appearance of the dental arch and reduce the signs of aging by adjusting centric and protrusive relationships, thinning edges, and recreating the anatomy and appearance of a more youthful tooth. In cases of significant loss of tooth structure, supported bonding, porcelain laminate veneers, or full-coverage porcelain restorations may be the treatment of choice.

Loss of facial enamel support causes the lip contour to hang lower on the tooth. The resulting decrease in the display of the incisal edge is a telltale sign of aging. When the facial surfaces of the maxillary anterior teeth are restored to their normal dimension and position, or the incisal edge is restored or increased, the patient's smile will take on a more youthful appearance. Full lip support reduces wrinkles and creasing around the lips and in the nasolabial fold areas of the face. It can even appear as if the patient has had a face lift.

Posterior teeth also lose their cuspal inclines slowly with wear. But this process is significantly accelerated with habits such as bruxism, clenching, and chewing on hard objects (*eg*, pens, pipes, popcorn kernels, ice, and hard candies). As these dimensions are lost, the face may take on a collapsed appearance. The loss of canine guidance will cause the posterior wear to occur at a faster rate. Increasing the vertical dimension with a full occlusal night guard can soften wrinkles and decrease the puckering of the face. The guard is a useful diagnostic tool in determining the goals of a treatment plan. In the case of an edentulous patient, the bite rim should be used to restore lost vertical dimension and drooping facial contours.

Surface texture, which affects the refraction, reflection, and absorption of light, slowly changes with age and a person's cleaning habits. Overaggressive use of a toothbrush, excessive amounts of abrasives in toothpaste, and inappropriate use of bleaches and cleansers can age a tooth in a very short time. Stripping of the facial enamel is likely to occur on the maxillary anterior teeth. Patients tend to focus on these teeth with the goal of brushing away stains and debris to keep their teeth white and their smiles bright. This aggressiveness in home care frequently results in a flatter surface texture and a change in the light-reflecting ability of the teeth. Patients rarely know that they are causing damage to their dentition. Counseling them on the minimal use of toothpaste, the use of a soft or ultrasoft brush, and the modification of brushing techniques is the best way to retard this process.

Maintenance techniques

As persons age, their ability to perform routine home care deteriorates. Their vision may become impaired. Their manual dexterity may be compromised by arthritis, stiffening of the joints, or loss of flexibility. Multiple-implement cleaning systems (such as the routine floss, brush, and rubber tip regimen) may become difficult and cumbersome, resulting in increasing bouts with periodontal disease and recurrent decay. Saliva and hormones are constantly modified by body chemistry throughout life and may cause alterations in host resistance factors. By understanding the patient's limitations and needs, the dentist may create office and home hygiene systems to aid in long-term maintenance.

Changes in office treatment include the introduction of piezoelectric scalers. Not only are these scalers more comfortable for the patient because of their linear motion, but they are able to reach difficult areas that might otherwise require hand scaling. The cavitation and irrigating effects of these scaling devices debride the root surfaces, leaving a smooth surface that is more resistant to plaque.

Neutral sodium gels, 1.1%, can be used in the office and dispensed for home use to increase tooth hardness and reduce the propensity for root caries. They are particularly beneficial to patients with significant root exposure or multiple restorative margins located on cementum; mouth breathers; those undergoing radiation, chemotherapy, or periodontal surgery; and those with root sensitivity. The new-generation bonding materials can also cover and protect the teeth, but only time will tell as to their longevity and effects on hypersensitivity.

Antibiotic cords are now being used to treat site-specific areas of periodontal involvement. This procedure reduces the overall systemic effect of the antibiotic and decreases the possibility of infection with antibiotic-resistant organisms. It allows the general dentist to treat the disease process aggressively in isolated areas where the patient may have difficulty cleaning and develops recurrent periodontal problems.

With the advent of new restorative materials, patients are becoming aware of the adverse effects of acids, alcohol, abrasives, acidulated and stannous fluorides, and habits that accelerate breakdown and wear. Special attention is given to concise postoperative instruction, which aids in minimizing problems and maintaining the restorations. Home care now focuses on the separation of and distinction between plaque removal and toothbrushing. Biofeedback mechanisms of plaque disorganization help the patient to appreciate this distinction.

"Re-care" or continuing care appointments should be scheduled at intervals to minimize the build-up of hard and soft debris, reduce the likelihood of periodontal progression, maintain the vitality and luster of the restored dentition, and aid the patient in the home hygiene regime. A 90-day re-care cycle has been found to be the most effective.

Conclusions

The aging population is now with us and will become a larger segment of our patient population for many years to come. To serve this population's needs to the best of our clinical and esthetic abilities, it will be necessary to understand the psychologic and physiologic changes that affect it. Tooth and facial aging, nutrition, and patient desires and resistance will affect our treatment decisions. This perspective, added to new scientific techniques, will help us better serve this population both functionally and esthetically.

Recommended reading

Papers of particular interest, published within the annual period of review, have been highlighted as:
- • Of special interest
- •• Of outstanding interest

1. Goldstein RE: **Esthetic dentistry: a health service?** [editorial]. *J Dent Res* 1993, 72:641–642.

2. Sheets CG: **Modern dentistry and the esthetically aware patient.** *J Am Dent Assoc,* 1987 Special issue:103E–105E.

3. Koury ME, Epker BN: **The aged face: the facial manifestations of aging.** *Int J Adult Orthod* 1991, 6:81–95.

4. Ofstehage J: **The social and psychological importance of dental-facial attractiveness in the elderly.** *Veterans Administration Newsletter* 1987, 1:31–33.

5. Adamson PA, Moran ML: **Historical trends in surgery for the aging face.** *Facial Plast Surg* 1993, 9:133–142.

6. Iacopino AM, Wathen WF: **Geriatric prosthodontics: part I. pretreatment considerations.** *Quintessence Int* 1993, 24:259–266.
••
Discusses psychologic aspects of aging and age-related changes in teeth, oral tissues, nutrition, and metabolism.

7. Iacopino AM, Wathen WF: **Geriatric prosthodontics: part I. Treatment considerations.** *Quintessence Int* 1993, 24:259–266.
••
Reviews restorative treatments for geriatric patients with caries, tooth wear, or missing teeth.

8. Douglass CW, Jette AM, Fox CH, Tennstedt SL, Joshi A, Feldman HA, McGuire SM, McKinlay JB: **Oral Health Status of the elderly in New England.** *J Gerontol* 1993, 3:M39–M46.
••
Reports on the prevalence, extent, and severity of oral diseases and conditions among the elderly population of New England and suggests that disease prevalence and severity may have been underreported in previous national surveys.

9. Newton JP, Yemm R, Abel RW, Menhinick S: **Changes in human jaw muscles with age and dental state.** *Gerodontology* 1993, 10:16–22.
•
Examines the effects of aging and dental state on the cross-sectional area and density of the masseter and medial pterygoid muscles. Changes in these muscles appeared to be consistent with age-related changes in muscle tissue throughout the body.

10. Jeffcoat MK, Chestnut CH: **Systemic osteoporosis and oral bone loss: evidence shows increased risk factors.** *J Am Acad Dent* 1993, 124:49–55.
•
Discusses risks of oral and systemic bone loss associated with aging. Topics covered include tooth loss and ridge resorption.

11. Newton JP, McManus FC: **The maintenance of oral function in the elderly.** *J Dent Res* 1991, 70:323.

12. Dolan TA, McNaughton CA, Davidson SN, Mitchell GS: **Patient Age and the general dentist's treatment decisions.** *Special Care Dent* 1992, 12:15–22.

13. Ettinger RL: **Restoring the aging dentition: repair or replacement?** *Int Dent J* 1990, 40:285–282.

14. Titus HW: **Root caries: some facts and treatment methods.** *J Am Dent Assoc* 1991, 4:61–68.

15. Mount GJ: **Restoration of eroded areas.** *J Am Dent Assoc* 1990, 120:31..35.

16. Shaecken MJ, Keltjens HM, Van Der Hoeven JS: **Effects of fluoride and chlorhexidine on the microflora of dental root surfaces and progression of root-surface caries.** *J Dent Res* 1991, 70:150–153.

Jacqueline Dzierzak, DMD, 626 North Michigan Avenue, Chicago, IL 60611, USA.

Methods and materials for porcelain veneers

Debra Gray King, DDS

Atlanta, Georgia, USA

Porcelain veneers are an esthetic, relatively conservative restoration used to cover the facial surface of the teeth. Following proper guidelines, the practitioner can achieve successful results as a matter of routine. This article reviews the most current literature published on this subject to bring practitioners up to date on clinical methods and materials used for porcelain veneers.

Porcelain veneers are custom-made shells of porcelain bonded to the facial surface of teeth. They are used to correct such esthetic deficiencies as chips or fractures of anterior teeth, interproximal spaces, color defects, and malaligned teeth. Accordingly, porcelain veneers can change the size of a tooth or the contour of a smile (Figs. 1 and 2) [1••,2••].

Preparation and pretreatment considerations

Concepts regarding the preparation of teeth for porcelain veneers have changed over the past few years. Although early concepts suggested minimal or no tooth preparation, current beliefs support removal of varying amounts of tooth structure [1••,3••,4•,5]. On one end of the spectrum, when the anterior teeth present relatively flat labial contours or are in linguoversion (*ie*, if porcelain is to be added to the facial aspect of the teeth to produce the effect of having the teeth moved facially), only the aprismatic layer of enamel needs to be removed [6••], not to allow room for the porcelain, but rather to improve the bonding strength.

The typical amount of reduction varies, however, from a minimum of 0.5 mm, which allows only for the thickness of the porcelain, to 0.75 mm, depending on the position of the tooth in the arch, to 1.0 mm, which would be necessary to mask a dark color of the underlying tooth structure. The most common amount of tooth reduction, between 0.5 and 0.75 mm [1••,3••,4•], is recommended for several reasons: 1) It avoids overcontouring [4•,5,6••–8••]; 2) it improves the color-masking properties of the veneer [1••,4•,8••]; 3) it improves the bond to the enamel [4•]; 4) it allows sufficient thickness of porcelain at the margins to resist chipping [4•]; and 5) it aids seating by including the incisal edge in the preparation [4•].

Regardless of the extent of reduction, certain shaping guidelines are similar. For example, all incisal angles should be rounded [4•,7••], and there should be no undercuts [2••,4•,6••]. Moreover, a chamfer-type labial preparation is strongly recommended for full-contour anterior teeth [3••] because it allows enough porcelain thickness for strength [1••]. If additional incisal length is needed, some form of wrap design is unavoidable [7••]. Furthermore, a slight separation should be obtained interproximally [4•,7••] to promote a clearer impression and assist the laboratory technician in determining where each veneer should begin. To this end, coarse finishing strips are ideal.

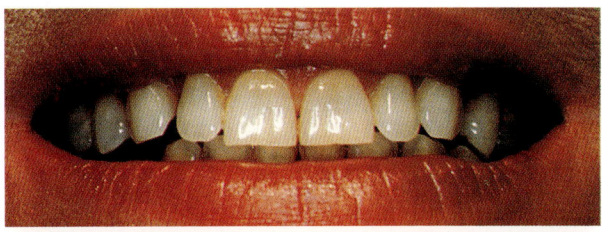

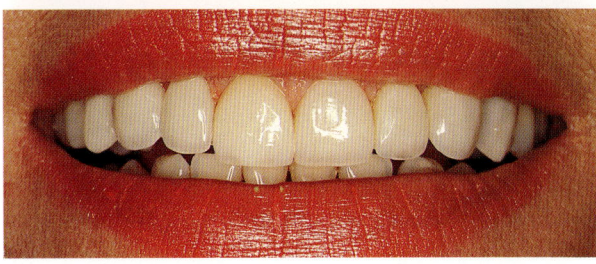

Fig. 1. Top, Preoperative photograph of patient who desired esthetic improvement. **Bottom,** The same patient after porcelain veneers were placed on the maxillary eight anterior teeth.

There are three basic preparation techniques for porcelain veneers: the common, the slice, and the window [2••]. Often, all three methods are used in the same case (Fig. 3).

The common preparation

The common preparation is the type most frequently recommended in current literature [1••,6••]. This type of preparation reduces facial tooth structure by approximately 0.5 mm, unless the teeth are especially dark

46 Cosmetic dentistry

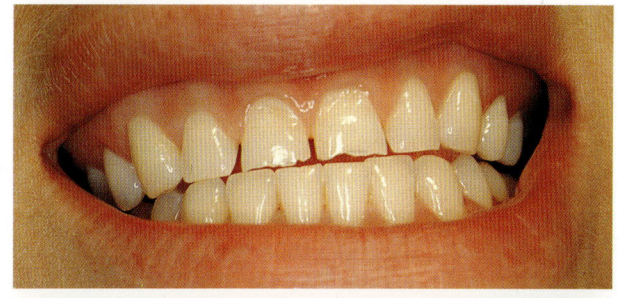

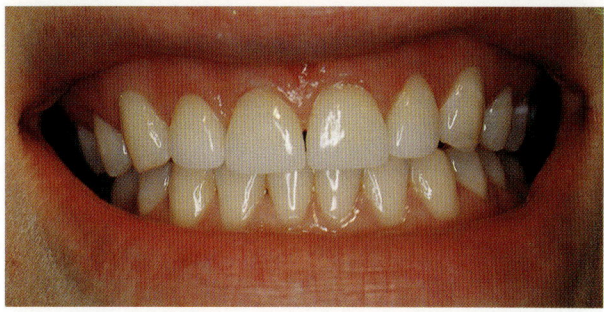

Fig. 2. Top, Preoperative photograph of a patient requiring cosmetic dentistry. **Bottom,** The same patient after porcelain veneers were placed on four maxillary incisors to close spaces and replace chipped incisal edges.

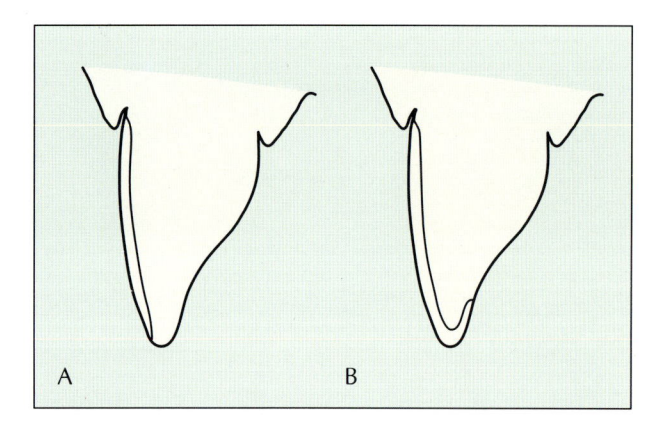

Fig. 3. A, Window preparation for porcelain application of laminate. **B,** Common preparation with overlapped incisal edge. (*Modified from* Gilmour and Stone [4•].)

and require more reduction (then, up to 1.0 mm) [2••]. This preparation is kept slightly superior to the gingival margin. Reduction extends into the interproximal areas anterior to the contact area, allowing only the prepared tooth structure to be viewed from any angle [1••,4•,6••]. When changes in the incisal edge are necessary, is then reduced by approximately 0.5 to 1.0 mm [2••,6••], as a reverse bevel or chamfer, without any sharp areas [1••,2••]. Great care is required with the occlusal contacts, especially in excursive movements [4•]. In addition, the incisal edge should be covered to prevent postoperative fractures, especially on the canines [3••]. The lingual porcelain material enhances the resistance to the facial forces on the veneer [6••]. Protrusive movement should not shear the bond, because the opposing incisors will come to contact with the porcelain, compressing it against the chamfer [6••,9].

The slice preparation

The slice preparation is used when it is necessary to close diastemata or to move the position of contact laterally from one tooth to the adjacent tooth, thereby effectively changing the size of the tooth [1••,2••]. The only significant difference between the common and the slice preparation is that the slice preparation continues lingually in the interproximal area, so that the contours of the porcelain veneer blend into the contours of lingual tooth structure [1••,2••].

The window preparation

The window preparation is also similar to the common preparation with modification at the incisal edge. A diamond bur commonly used to place a chamfer is turned upside down, and the cut is made from the facial surface at the incisal edge so that the angle of the incisal-facial line is not altered [1••,2••].

The window preparation method has a number of notable disadvantages. It requires strong tooth structure at the incisal edge and may not withstand excessive forces from bruxism or parafunctional habits [1••,2••].

Furthermore, if teeth are prepared on the facial surface only, the incisal edge will be weakened and fragile [6••]. Cementation can be more difficult without an aid to seating, and the incisal margin finished in the translucent tip of the tooth can give an inferior esthetic result [4•]. Therefore, the window preparation is not routinely used. The most recent theories involve preparing the incisal edge in all cases and placing a lingual chamfer [6••].

Beginning the procedure

Because of the reduction in the enamel, local anesthetic is generally necessary. Short-duration, 3% mepivicaine without vasoconstrictor is usually adequate [3••].

A diamond bur should be used to keep the preparation in enamel, if possible, and the amount of tooth structure is reduced according to the previously discussed criteria. The amount of tooth reduction can be monitored with a Brasseler 834-021 diamond bur (Brasseler USA, Savannah, GA) for depth cuts, and a 843-023 bur may be used to complete the gross reduction. Another method is to use a diamond bur with a 0.5-mm diameter and to make depth cuts at this width vertically along the facial surface to gauge the amount of enamel that will be removed. It is important to keep the margins of the preparation in enamel, because retaining porcelain veneer margins to etched enamel prevents microleakage [1••,4•,7••]. Some microleakage is observed when margins are terminated on a dentinal surface, regardless of the dentin bonding agents used [7••].

To obtain slight retraction, a thin, nonmedicated retraction cord may be placed in the gingival sulcus from the distal papilla across the facial area to the mesial papilla [3••, 6••]. The cord will allow the preparation to extend further apically and will limit seepage of the sulcular fluid [8••]. Leave the cord in place during the impression and fabrication of provisional veneers. Beautiful results may also be obtained by placing the prepared margin immediately at the gingival margin without the use of a retraction cord. Whether to use a cord is simply the clinician's choice.

Shade selection

It is important to involve the patient with the shade selection. The final shade of the veneers depends not only on the shade of the porcelain but also on the color of the underlying tooth and of the composite luting cement [4•]. If only the maxillary arch is being done, it is not always necessary to match the color to a dark lower arch. The patient will usually appreciate teeth at least a few shades lighter, and it is not uncommon naturally to have slightly darker lower teeth. This choice also allows the patient, if he or she wishes, to choose to veneer the lower teeth at a future date. More important, porcelain veneers do not all have to be the same shade. In fact, to obtain a more realistic result, the veneers should vary in color as natural shading. If the most posterior unprepared tooth is slightly darker than the patient prefers, ask the laboratory technician to blend the porcelain to a lighter shade towards the anterior. For example, if the premolars are shade A3, have the laboratory prepare the distal area of the canines in shade A3, the mesial section of the canines and distal area of the lateral incisors in A2, and the mesial area of the lateral incisors and the entire central incisors in A1. Also consider whitening the posterior teeth with an at-home whitening system such as Nite White (Discus Dental, Beverly Hills, CA) or Opalescence (Ultradent Products, Salt Lake City, UT) prior to shade selection. Complete the whitening process at least 2 weeks before seating the veneers so as not to interfere with the bond. Detailed communication with the laboratory technician regarding shade and contour is extremely important.

Impression

Impressions for veneers, if done correctly, can be simple, fast, and accurate. If a retraction cord was used, leave it in place during the impression. A double-arch impression tray is adequate in many cases [3••], although many clinicians still prefer full-arch impressions.

Even when the preparation is slightly subgingival, retraction may not be necessary to get a good impression. Placing the syringe at the margin of the preparation and forcing the impression material subgingivally will result in an enhanced impression defining the subgingival margin [2••]. If margins are definitive and properly registered in the final impression, the veneers should fit the preparations precisely [10].

Impression materials include the following [3••]:

1. Exaflex (G-C America, Chicago, IL)

2. Express (3M Dental Products, St. Paul, MN)

3. Extrude (Kerr Manufacturing Co., Romulus, MI)

4. Permagum (Premier Dental Products, Norristown, PA)

5. Reprosil (Dentsply International, LD Caulk Division, Milford, DE)

6. Cutter (Miles, South Bend, IN)

Temporization

Temporization is the choice of the practitioner and is occasionally bypassed to allow the patient to clean the area properly. The practitioner should note, however, that temporization is time-consuming and adds considerable cost to the procedure [5]. If minor amounts of reduction are made, and the teeth are not uncomfortably sensitive, no temporization is necessary. As an alternate approach to temporization, sensitivity of exposed dentin can be avoided by applying five to 10 layers of dentinal bonding agents to the unetched tooth surface [2••].

When temporization is required because of tooth sensitivity or the patient's esthetic concerns, several material options exist, including composite or acrylic resins. When several teeth are involved, an esthetic result can be obtained by using a vacuum-formed splint made from preoperative study models with acrylic resin. To maximize strength, keep all teeth connected. Petroleum jelly should be applied to the teeth to allow easy removal. Acrylic burs and disks can then be used to open embrasure areas and adjust contours. The veneers can be cemented in place with Durelon cement (Premier Dental Products, Norristown, PA) or bonded with a thin reline layer of acrylic [2••].

When temporization of one or two teeth is necessary, or if the best esthetic outcome is desired, composite resin is the material of choice. The tooth should be spot-etched on the center of the facial surface and the composite molded onto the prepared tooth. The composite can be contoured to the required shape and

48 Cosmetic dentistry

the marginal and interproximal areas thinned for easy cleaning prior to curing. This process is similar to direct composite veneering or free-hand veneering, and with practice can be completed in a very short time. Frequently, the only adjustment needed is on the incisal edge, and so removal of the temporary veneer is not necessary until the insertion appointment [2••]. This method will give the best esthetic and retentive result. With any type of temporization, it is important to limit the patient to a soft diet and advise the patient that the temporary veneer may loosen.

Placement

Anesthetize the area if necessary. Thoroughly clean the teeth with pumice and water or the prophy jet. Try in each porcelain veneer individually, then collectively with try-in paste. After patient and dentist approval, the veneers are ready to be prepared for placement.

Place the veneers in a beaker of distilled water and clean them with an ultrasonic cleaner [2••]. Keep in mind that failure is usually caused by contamination of one or both bonding surfaces during placement. Etch the internal surface of the veneer with a mild, diluted, 2% solution of hydrofluoric acid for 2 minutes to obtain a chalky white appearance [2••]. Apply several layers of silane and unfilled resin and then blow dry [2••,4•]. The silane will increase adhesion and reduce microleakage [11]. There seem to be no conclusive studies indicating clear superiority of one adhesive system over another. Each system has its own unique advantages and disadvantages. The clinician's choice depends on his or her own personal preference [11]. More important, the

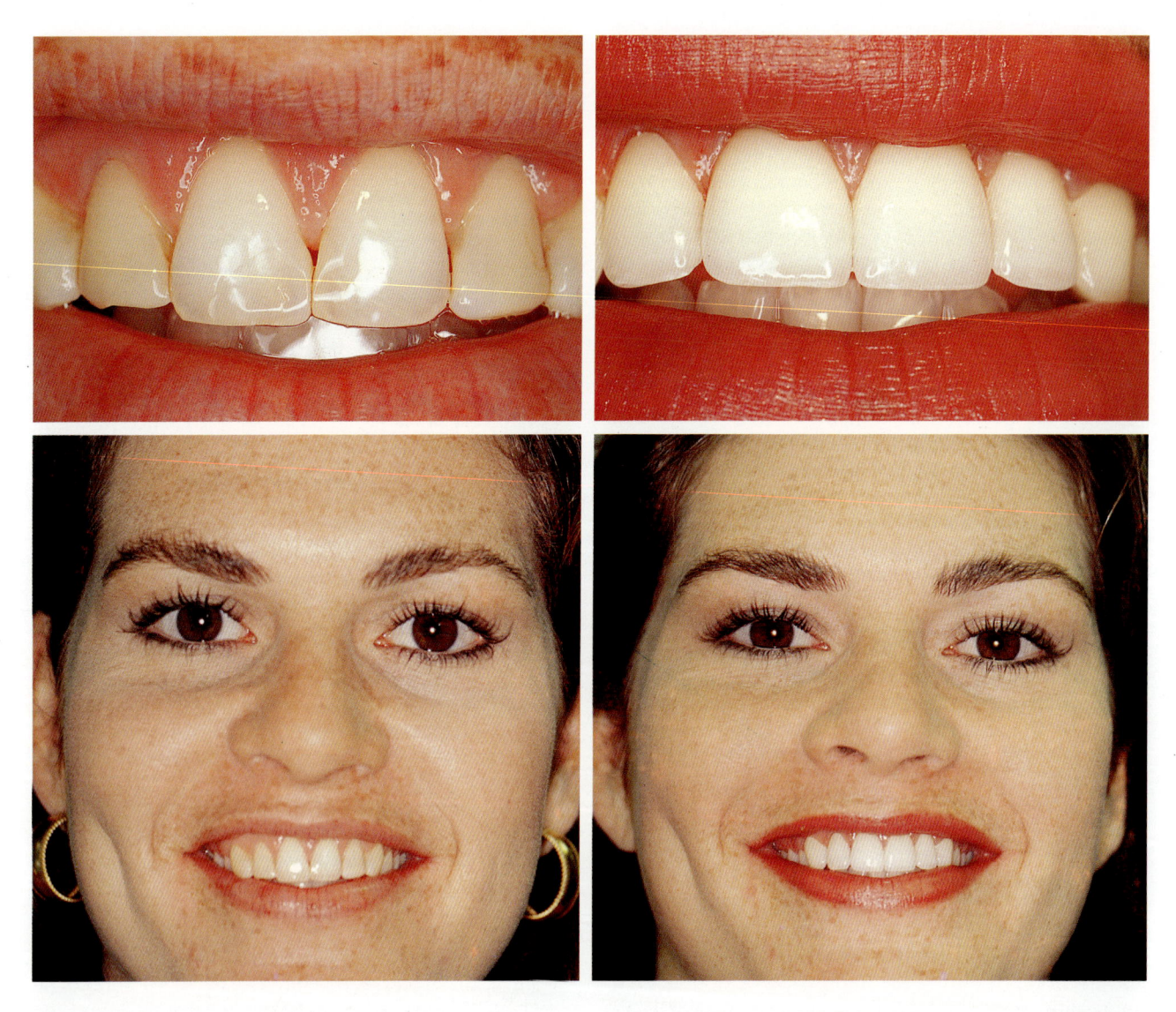

Fig. 4. Top left, Preoperative photograph of a patient's smile shows old composite filling and bonding. **Top right,** Postoperative photograph with porcelain veneers in place on teeth 6, 7, 8, 9, 10, and 11. **Bottom left,** Preoperative, full-face photograph of the same patient. **Bottom right,** Postoperative, full-face view.

practitioner must strictly adhere to the application protocol of the system chosen.

A few of the more popular bonding products include the following [3••]:

1. ABC (Chameleon Dental Products, Kansas City, KS)

2. All-Bond 2 (Bisco, Itasca, IL)

3. Scotchbond Multi-Purpose (3M Dental Products)

The teeth should be etched with a 37% solution of phosphoric acid for 15 seconds [1••]. Avoid etching the adjacent teeth by placing a Mylar strip (Du Pont Co., Wilmington, DE) around the lingual of the tooth [3••]. Rinse thoroughly. Apply several coats of a chlorhexidine gluconate cleaner and dry [2••]. Follow with five to 10 layers of dentinal bonding agents and air-dry. Apply a thin layer of unfilled bonding resin but do not cure. Keep the overhead light off to prevent early polymerization. [2••] Take care to avoid resin pooling in the sites of the intersection of the planes with a gentle spray of air [9].

Popular cements for veneers include the following [3••]:

1. Heliolink (Ivoclar North America, Amherst, NY)

2. Indirect Porcelain System (3M Dental Products)

3. Insure (Cosmedent, Chicago, IL)

4. Mirage FLC (Chameleon Dental Products)

5. Porcelite (Kerr Manufacturing Co.)

6. Ultrabond (Den-Mat Corp., Santa Maria, CA)

Place the composite resin on the internal surface of the veneer and position it on the tooth. Begin with the central incisors and move posteriorly. It is important that the veneer be placed so that excess resin flows freely from the margins without entrapping air [1••,2••]. To prevent fracture, do not exert excessive pressure during placement [1••]. A recent study showed that using a fine brush moistened with a bonding agent to remove composite resin before polymerization may well reduce marginal integrity by diluting the filler content of the luting composite [7••]. Instead, remove excess resin with cotton swabs and an explorer. Leave a small amount of excess resin at edges of the veneer.

Cure from the lingual side of the tooth for 60 seconds. Because filled resin shrinks in the direction of the light beam, there may be a more intimate resin-enamel contact with initial through-the-tooth curing [8••]. Cure from the facial surface for an additional 60 seconds. Regardless of the thickness or opacity of the veneer, the presence of the veneer will double the setting time of the composite resins beneath it [7••]. Light activation alone will cure veneers of varying opacity levels with average thickness of 0.7 mm [7••]

Thickness ranges of 1 mm need increased irradiation times to achieve adequate monomer conversion [7••]. Because composites cannot be overcured, double the recommended exposure time prior to finishing [7••]. Several dual-cure systems that produce greater degrees of cure and material hardness are available [7••].

After curing, excess cement can be removed with a Komet 150.32 hand instrument (Brasseler USA) or a no. 12 or no. 15 scalpel [10]. If hand instruments rather than rotary are used, the high luster of the glazed veneer will not be lost. If significant excess resin remains, use an 8, then a 16, then finally a 30 fluted carbide bur, until a small enough amount of resin remains to use the hand instrument for removal [1••,2••,6••]. Adjust the occlusion after checking for premature contacts with articulating paper. Interproximal margins require the use of finishing strips of decreasing abrasiveness to remove any overhangs [4•].

Polish with points or rubber wheels where needed. Diamond and polishing-cone finishing should be completed with a water coolant to avoid the excessive heat that causes chipping at the porcelain margins [4•]. Very little polishing is needed, however, if only hand instruments are used to remove the excess resin.

The patient should be cautioned that the first 2 hours after placing the porcelain veneers are the most critical. The patient should avoid medium-consistency to hard foods, alcohol, and acid liquids such sodas or citrus juices [12]. The patient should begin with a soft diet and then gradually over the next 3 to 4 days use these teeth more while biting and chewing. This graduation will minimize any excessive stresses that could potentially chip or fracture the veneers [12].

After the first few days, the patient can chew normally on the veneers, although he or she should continue to avoid extremely hard material such as ice, hard candies, corn kernels, apples, or carrots. Bad habits like clenching, grinding, and biting on pencils or fingernails should be discouraged [12].

Conclusions

Porcelain veneers have revolutionized the treatment of esthetic problems of anterior teeth. Although the procedure requires great concentration and precision, the clinician can achieve restorations that closely resemble natural dentition while conserving tooth structure (Fig. 4).

Acknowledgment

I would like to acknowledge the dental technicians at Masterworks International of Atlanta, Georgia.

References and recommended reading

Papers of particular interest, published within the annual period of review, have been highlighted as:
- Of special interest
- • Of outstanding interest

1. •• Chalifoux, PR: **Porcelain Veneers.** *Curr Opin Cosmetic Dent* 1994, 2:58–66.

The author presents a thorough and up-to-date review of the techniques important for successful porcelain veneer restorations.

2. •• Chalifoux PR, Darvish M: **Porcelain veneers: concept, preparation, temporization, laboratory, and placement.** *Pract Periodontics Aesthet Dent* 1993, 5:11–17.

This article presents a detailed and comprehensive review of the techniques necessary for the preparation and cementation of porcelain veneers.

3. •• **Porcelain veneer update 1993.** *Clinical Research Associates Newsletter* 1993, 17(6).

This short article presents concise and specific details that allow the clinician to produce porcelain veneers from start to finish. It also includes recommended materials.

4. • Gilmour ASM, Stone DC: **Porcelain laminate veneers: a clinical success?** *Dent Update* 1993, 20:167–169, 171–173.

This article describes pretreatment considerations, types of preparations, laboratory procedures, and causes of failure.

5. Jordan RE: **Aesthetic composite bonding techniques and materials.** In *Aesthetic Composite Bonding*. Philadelphia: BC Decker; 1987.

6. •• Chpindel, P, Cristou M: **Tooth preparation and fabrication of porcelain veneers using a double-large technique.** *Pract Periodontics Aesthet Dent* 1994, 6:19–30.

This is a fully illustrated, comprehensive article that should aid the practitioner in achieving consistently excellent clinical results.

7. •• Friedman MJ: **Current state-of-the-art porcelain veneers.** *Curr Opin Cosmetic Dent* 1993, 1:28–33.

This article presents an interesting investigation of the clinical and scientific issues pertaining to determine the parameters for efficacy.

8. •• Cavanaugh RR, Croll TP: **Bonded porcelain veneer-masking of dark tetracycline dentinal stains.** *Pract Periodontics Aesthet Dent* 1994, 6:71–79.

This case presentation describes in detail current techniques and includes step-by-step illustrations for successful porcelain veneer restorations.

9. Harster P, Martinez J: **Lingually-reverted laminate veneers: clinical procedure and case presentation.** *Pract Periodontics Aesthet Dent* 1993, 5:57–64.

10. Miller, MB: **Aesthetic anterior reconstruction using a combined periodontal/restorative approach.** *Pract Periodontics Aesthet Dent* 1993, 5:33–40.

11. Jackson RD: **Esthetic inlays and onlays.** *Curr Opin Cosmetic Dent* 1994, 2:30–39.

12. Dzierzak J: *Form 6004*. Chicago: Subtle Impressions.

Debra Gray King, DDS, 4840 Roswell Road, Building A, Atlanta, GA 30342, USA.

Indirect composite restorations

William G. Dickerson, DDS, and James H. Hastings, DDS

Las Vegas, Nevada, and Placerville, California, USA

The evolution of composite and adhesive technology has benefited dentistry significantly. The 1990s have brought us, for the first time in the history of our profession, the ability to restore tooth structure in a conservative and esthetic fashion. The ability to give consistently high-bond strengths to both enamel and dentin and the excellent physical properties of these restorations have made them a permanent part of restorative dentistry. This paper summarizes the authors' current opinion about indirect composite restorations, outlines indications for their use, and describes a clinical technique for their preparation and cementation.

The indirect composite restoration was developed to serve as a predictable esthetic restorative, a compromise between amalgam or direct composite, which can fill small cavities in posterior teeth, and gold onlays or full-coverage porcelain crowns, which require removal of most enamel and often sound dentin [1••]. Some of the problems with silver amalgam are marginal leakage, inadequate strength, weakening of the tooth, incompatible co-efficient of thermal expansion, a wear rate different from that of the natural tooth structure, and the continuing controversy that the silver amalgam filling contains about 50% mercury upon initial placement, which is released into the body. In addition, silver amalgam is unsightly when placed in the mouth, and because it expands as it ages, it is frequently implicated as the cause of occult or frank fractures of the tooth it originally saved from decay. Because of these negative characteristics, an alternative to the amalgam restoration has been sought for years.

Direct composite materials have improved considerably in the past few years. Wear rates can be similar to those of amalgam and approach those of natural enamel [2]. There are also problems associated with the direct composite, however. Polymerization shrinkage, which in turn can cause gap formation, microleakage, and pulpal sensitivity, is the greatest drawback to its use in large restorations. In addition, it is a challenge to restore proximal contact and contour and to create a gingival seal with the direct composite. Many writers have addressed these issues, using a variety of techniques [3]. No matter which technique was used, it took significant time and skill to restore teeth requiring replacement of more than a small amount of their original structure. These challenges are commonly labeled *technique sensitivity*.

The indirect composite overcomes all of the drawbacks associated with the other two restorative materials. Shrinkage takes place in the laboratory and is controlled by the technician. The contours and contacts are established by the technician before the restoration is brought to the mouth. The indirect composite requires additional practice for consistent results, but the results that can be obtained are nothing short of esthetically spectacular when compared with those obtained with silver amalgam (Figs. 1 and 2), gold, or porcelain-to-metal technology. The time and dedication needed to become proficient in the use of the indirect composite restoration are well worth the effort in terms of patient satisfaction and satisfaction for the clinician. Although exacting, the technique is not difficult, if care is taken and attention is paid to detail.

The introduction of the "fourth-generation" bonding agents has allowed the indirect composite restoration to be used confidently. With bond strengths approaching or exceeding that of enamel to dentin, the clinician can now place a restoration in the truest sense of the word, *ie*, one that replaces the original form, function, and appearance of the natural tooth.

Although the esthetic qualities of this restoration are the most striking initially, the physical properties are remarkable as well. The wear against natural enamel is the most like that of enamel itself [4]. The reproduction of lifelike anatomy, the ability to produce seamless margins, conservation of natural tooth structure, and the near restoration

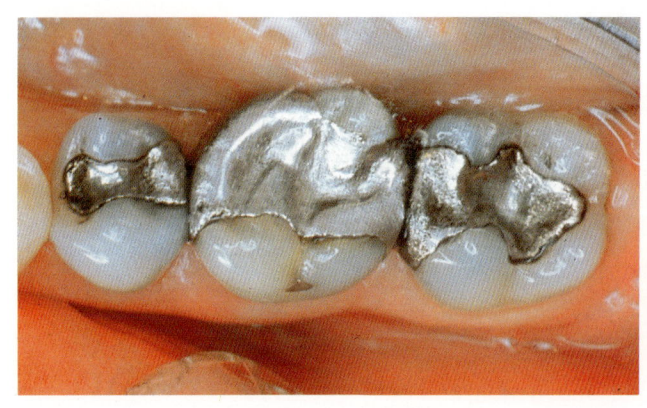

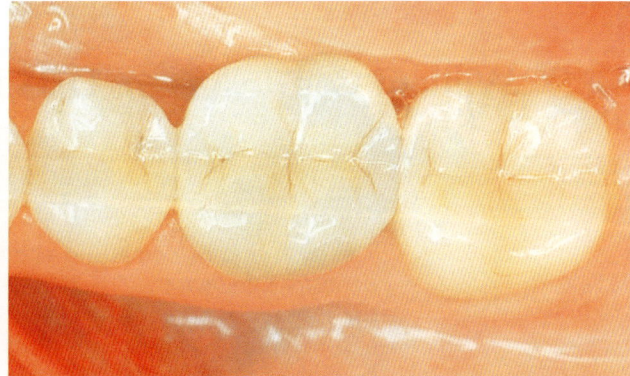

Fig. 1. Left, Quadrant of amalgams before replacement. **Right,** Quadrant of indirect resin replacements.

of the original strength of the damaged tooth are qualities that have made the indirect composite a significant part of the armamentarium of a number of restorative dentists [5,6,7••,8].

Properties

Numerous manufacturers are producing composite materials that can be used in this application. Most are hybrid materials, with an average inorganic filler particle size of 0.7 to 4 µm. All except one are cured by light; in some, heat treating follows the curing of restoration. The one exception, Concept (Ivoclar-Williams, Amherst, NY), uses a combination of heat and pressure to cure. Concept is a microfill with 76% inorganic filling by weight. This inorganic loading is greater than that possible with direct microfill composites. The high temperature (125°C) used in treating the material produces nearly an 85% conversion in polymerization, higher than is available with any other system [9] (Rueggeberg, Personal communication). The pressure curing at 80 psi eliminates voids found with indirect or other direct systems. The small and uniform particle size (0.4 µm) lends itself best to polishability and the reproduction of a lifelike esthetic quality. The heat and pressure curing provide an increase in flexural strength, surface hardness, and polymerization as well as a reduction in solubility [10]. Because of these enhanced physical properties, another manufacturer is close to releasing a heat- and pressure-cured system of its own and may have already done so at the time of this publication. An added benefit of Concept is a radiopacifying agent that releases fluoride and has been shown to reduce caries around the restorations [11,12].

Indications and use

At the time of this writing, we have placed several thousand of these restorations in many different situations. We believe that it can be used in all areas of the mouth, depending on the size of the restoration in molars.

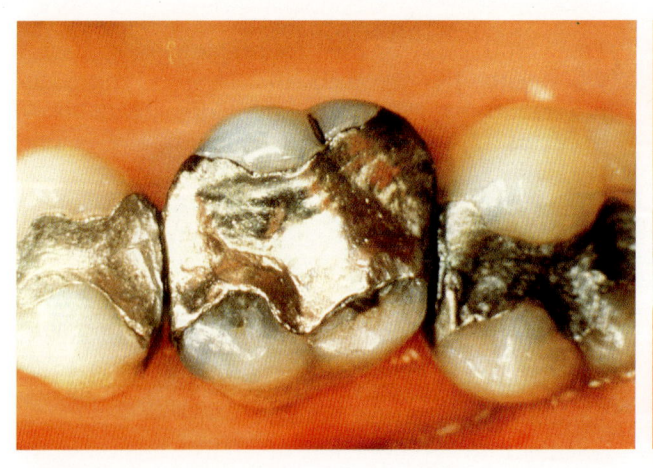

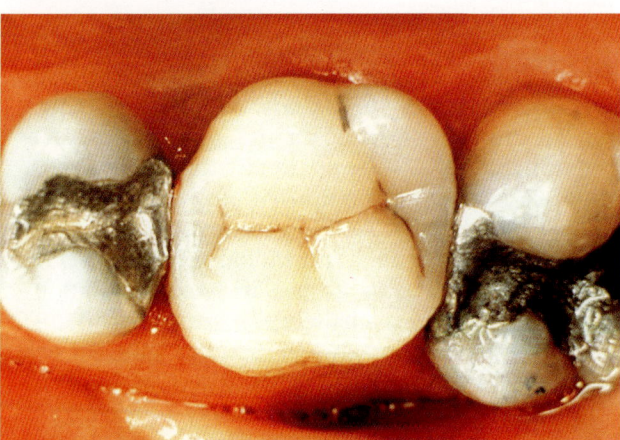

Fig. 2. Left, A very large amalgam with thin buccal and lingual walls remaining. **Right,** Indirect resin restoration without the need for cuspal coverage.

Range of application

As clinicians have gained experience with the use of indirect composites, they have proven beneficial in a wide range of applications including cusp replacement, full coverage, post-core and crown, and short-span posterior and anterior bridges [13,14] (Hornbrook, Personal communication). The maxillary anterior bridge usually requires a porcelain veneer on the pontic for best esthetic results.

Ease of use

The technique for the indirect composite is significantly different from that of the conventional crown and bridge. New techniques require additional training and experience, but they are within the reach of any practitioner willing to learn. Clinicians experienced in the technique have found it to be easier overall than conventional crown and bridge, and far more satisfying to use. The following is a technique for preparation and insertion of the indirect composite restoration. Although this description involves materials specific to the Concept restoration, it can be applied to any brand of indirect composite.

Preparation

In preparing the tooth for the indirect composite, the following steps are taken:

1. The selected tooth is anesthetized, as necessary.

2. The shade is selected according to the system being used. The base shade is usually selected from the cervical third of the buccal surface to create a restoration with depth. The occlusal shade is translucent and picks up the color of the existing tooth.

3. The rubber dam is placed. Although placement is not mandatory for the preparation appointment, it is a good habit to get into, and it saves time in the long run.

4. Preparation is straightforward. All amalgam and decay are removed. An occlusal clearance of at least 1.5 mm is needed, with a 2-mm width at the isthmus. Rounded internal line angles and tapered internal walls are a must. Unsupported enamel and undercuts are best blocked out by placing a hybrid composite or resin and ionomer. Enamel left standing with minimal or no dentin support is susceptible to fracture at the removal of the temporary restoration or the seating of the final restoration. The cusp should be capped, or "shoed," in this situation.

5. Internal walls and floor are smoothed and finished with a diamond or bur.

6. Cord is packed, only if necessary, for a dry field or visibility of the margin.

7. The rubber dam is removed, and the final impression is taken. A polyvinyl siloxane material is preferred because it is repourable, and the laboratory needs at least two models for fabrication of the inlay or onlay.

8. Bite registration is taken.

9. The tooth is washed with chlorhexidine (Peridex 12%: Proctor & Gamble, Cincinnati, OH; or Consepsis 2.0%: Ultradent Products, Salt Lake City, UT) and dried without rinsing. This reduces or eliminates bacterial ingress into the dentinal tubules, a major cause of postoperative sensitivity. A light-cured temporary material is placed into the cavity preparation. The patient is asked to bite and grind. Excess material is re-

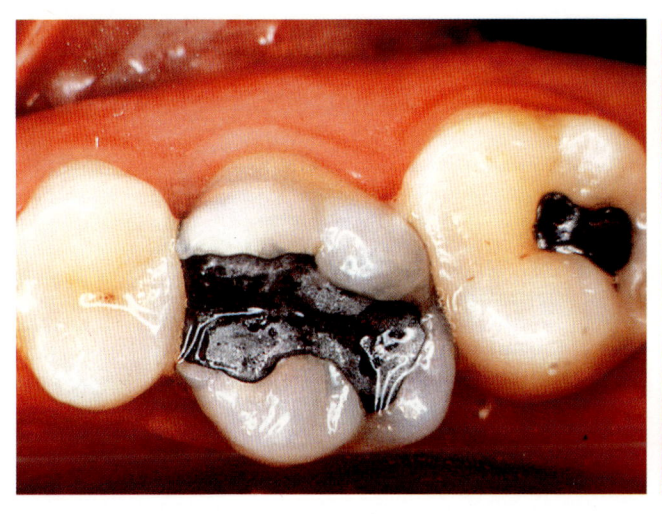

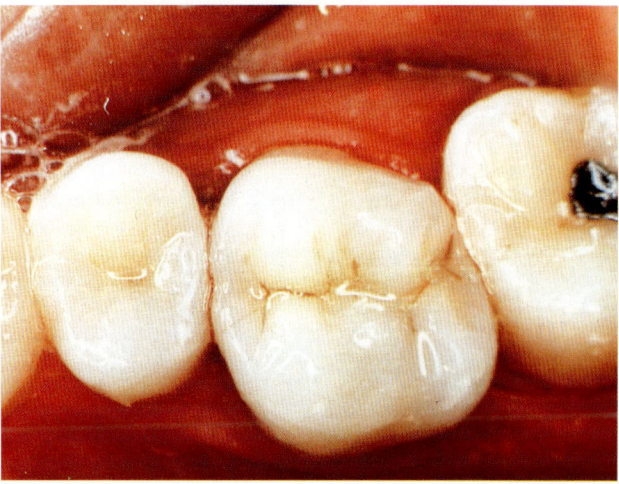

Fig. 3. Left, Dark amalgam before replacement with indirect resin. **Right,** Esthetic, functional, and tooth-supportive indirect resin restoration.

moved with hand instruments, and the patient should bite and grind again. The temporary restoration is light-cured for 20 seconds, and the occlusion checked. Any premature contacts can be removed with coarse diamonds or large round burs. This temporary material is flexible; sensitivity may be a problem if the material is in premature contact. It is a quick and easy temporary material to place, and removal and clean-up are simple. The temporary material is not cemented, because use of temporary cement has been shown to increase microleakage in the permanently bonded restorations [15].

Laboratory communication

The ability of the restoration to mimic natural tooth structure depends on the properties of the material and the accuracy with which the dentist communicates shade variations and stains to the technician. Knowledge of how enamel and dentin compose a natural tooth is helpful in building a lifelike final restoration [7••].

Cementation

In cementing the indirect composite, the following steps are taken:

1. The selected tooth is anesthetized, as necessary.

2. The rubber dam is placed. This is mandatory for moisture control and ease of composite placement. The bond strength is increased with use of the rubber dam [16], and much time and frustration are saved as well.

3. The temporary material is removed, and the preparation is cleaned with chlorhexidine. Chlorhexidine has antibacterial properties that may decrease postoperative sensitivity, and it has no effect on bond strength [17].

4. The tooth is dried, and the restoration is tried in. Marginal fit and quality of proximal contacts are assessed. The contact may be added to if necessary by sandblasting the contact area, applying silane if restoration is a hybrid or Special Bond II (Vivadent, Amherst, NY) if it is a microfill such as Concept. Place a thin layer of a luting composite, such as Dual Cement (Vivadent), to the etched area. This composite is cured with a light source, adjusted as necessary, and polished. Occlusal adjustment and final polish are done after cementation.

5. The internal surface is cleaned with a 37% phosphoric acid solution (only if contaminated from try-in), rinsed, and dried.

6. A matrix is placed in the interproximal area to avoid etching the adjacent tooth, and making final clean-up easier. Etch the tooth with a 30% to 40% phosphoric acid solution. It is best to place the etchant with a small cannula syringe for accurate placement. The enamel is etched first, including 1 mm of unprepared enamel surface, and then the dentin is etched. The total etching time is 15 seconds on the enamel and 10 seconds on the dentin. The etching demineralizes the dentin and creates a layer for the resin to penetrate and form the hybrid layer [18–20].

7. The prepared tooth is rinsed, lightly dried but not desiccated, and the matrix removed. A dentin moistening agent is applied to induce the hydrophilic primer to flow into the dentinal tubules. Tubulicid Red (Global Dental, North Bellmore, NY) is used because it contains benzalkonium chloride and sodium fluoride, 1.0%, which help to prevent caries and bacterial infection. We also use dexamethasone for its anti-inflamma-

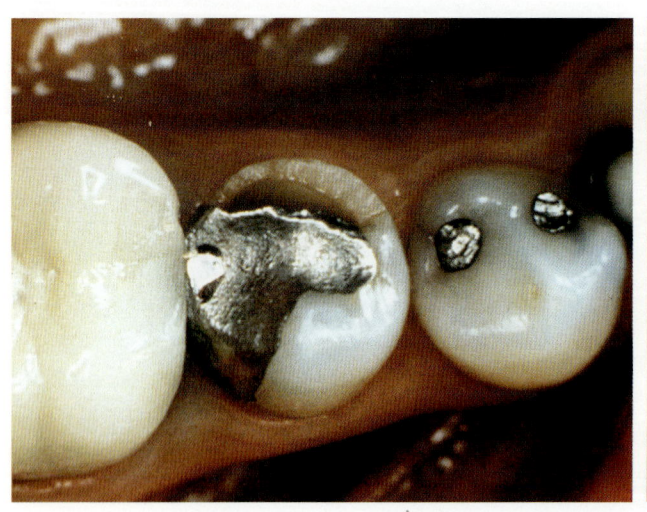

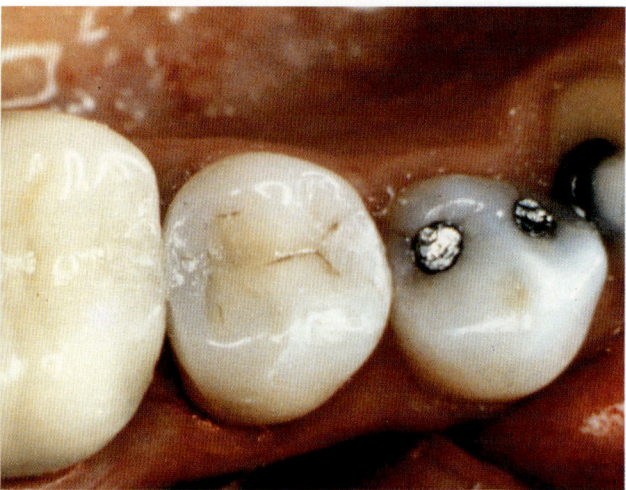

Fig. 4. *Left,* Large amalgam on the second bicuspid, the lingual cusp of which is fractured. *Right,* Conservative indirect resin replacement.

tory properties. Wetting the dentin has been proven to improve bond strength [21••].

8. Primer from a fourth-generation bonding agent is applied in several coats for about 30 seconds, then lightly air-dried to evaporate the solvent. It is imperative to use a hydrophilic bonding agent, because vital dentin will always be wet owing to the pulpal pressure and fluid in the tubules. The dentin surface should appear shiny, which indicates that the primer has sealed the dentinal tubules. Application of primer to the enamel has been shown to have no adverse effect on enamel bond strength [11].

9. A dentin bonding agent is applied to all surfaces, then thinned with a brush to prevent pooling of the resin. The resin is not light-cured at this time.

10. Special Bond II (for a microfill) or silane (for hybrids) is applied to the internal surface of the restoration, while the dual-cure cement is being mixed. A microfill dual-cure cement provides better polishability and wear resistance [22].

11. The cement is applied to the internal surface of the restoration, and the restoration is seated under the pressure of a blunt instrument, such as an acorn carver. Initial clean-up is done with a dry brush, rubber point, and explorer. The restoration is spot-cured with a 2-mm light guide for 10 seconds. Additional time is then spent in the removal of uncured cement. Floss is drawn through the contacts and across the margin area to remove excess cement. Thorough clean-up of excess cement is critical to expedient finishing later.

12. An oxygen barrier, such as De-Ox (Ultradent Dental Products) or Liquid Strip (Vivadent, Schaan, Liechtenstein) is applied to the margins to prevent formation of an oxygen inhibition layer and excess wear of the cement interface [22].

13. A large-diameter, high-intensity visible curing light is applied to the restoration. Curing through the tooth from the bucca and lingua simultaneously with two lights is recommended. With adequate light sources, 1 minute from each side and 1 minute from the occlusal side should be adequate for complete cure. Light sources should be routinely checked to ensure adequate output. Additional time should be added if the restoration is very large or deep.

14. Any additional resin flash is removed with scalers and rotating finishing burs or diamond instruments.

15. Remove the rubber dam and check the occlusion. Adjust the occlusion with finishing burs or diamonds. Check carefully for flash and remove. Use of the Profin (Weissman Technology, New York, NY) may be necessary interproximally if the initial clean-up was inadequate.

16. Polish the inlay with impregnated rubber polishing cups and points. Final polishing is done with a polishing paste, such as Prisma Gloss (Caulk Co., Milford, DE) or Enamelize (Cosmedent, Chicago, IL).

17. Rinse and dry the tooth and etch with phosphoric acid, 37% for 10 seconds. Dry and apply a surface sealer (Fortify; Bisco, Itasca, IL), and light-cure for 20 seconds. Rinse. Application of a surface sealer has been shown to seal the microfractures that occur in finishing and to increase the wear resistance of the restoration.

Conclusions

The indirect composite restoration is conservative, functionally sound, and tooth-supportive, as well as esthetically satisfying (Figs. 3 and 4). It can be used when a conventional crown might have been prescribed. Its inclusion in the restorative armamentarium has revitalized many practices, our own included. Patients are enthusiastic about the results, and the dentist has the satisfaction of creating a *true* restoration by returning the dentition to its natural form and function.

References and recommended reading

Papers of particular interest, published within the annual period of review, have been highlighted as:
- • Of special interest
- •• Of outstanding interest

1. •• Jackson R: **Esthetic inlays and onlays.** *Curr Opin Cosmetic Dent* 1994, 2:30–39.
A comprehensive effort to standardize the technique for preparation and delivery of any esthetic inlay or onlay system.

2. Bayne SC, Heymann HO, Swift EJ: **Update on dental composite restorations.** *J Am Dent Assoc* 1994, 125:687–701.

3. Crispin B, Hewlett E, Young HJ, Sumiya H, Hornbrook D: **Restorative esthetic procedures: direct composite and glass ionomer.** In *Contemporary Esthetic Dentistry: Practice Fundamentals*. Edited by Crispin BJ. Chicago: Quintessence Publishing Co.; 1994:132–134.

4. Burgoyne A, Nicholls J, Brudvik J: **In vitro two-body wear of inlay-onlay composite resin restoratives.** *J Prosthet Dent* 1991, 65:206–214.

5. Dickerson W: **Indirect resin restorations: all the benefits without the disadvantages.** *Dent Today* 1991, 10:32–36.

6. Dickerson W: **Indirect resin restoration: a proper technique to ensure success.** *Compendium* 1993, 14:216–224.

7. •• Jackson R: **Aesthetic inlays and onlays: a clinical technique update.** *Pract Periodontics Aesthet Dent* 1993, 5:18–26.
Describes a "generic color map" for laboratory communication that allows closer replication of natural tooth structure and more lifelike characteristics.

8. Shapiro J: **Achieving cosmetic and functional excellence with indirect resin inlays and onlays.** *Dent Econ* 1993, 83:88–89.

9. Freedman G, McLaughlin G: **Indirect composite restorative materials: a buyers guide.** *Dent Today* 1991, 10:30–32.

10. Gregory WA, Berry S, Duke E, Dennison JB: **Physical properties and repair bond strength of direct and indirect composite resins.** *J Prosthet Dent* 1992, 68:406–411.

11. Arends J, Ruben J, Dijkman A: **The effect of fluoride release from a fluoride-containing composite resin on secondary caries: an in vitro study.** *Quintessence Int* 1990, 21:671–674.

12. Ferracane JL, Condon JR: **Rate of elution of leachable components from composite.** *Dent Mater* 1990, 6:282–287.

13. Dickerson W: **A conservative alternate to single tooth replacement: a three year follow-up.** *Pract Periodontics Aesthet Dent* 1993, 5:43–48.

14. Dickerson W: **An aesthetic, conservative reconstruction technique for an endodontically prepared tooth.** *Quintessence Int* 1991, 2:935–938.

15. Woody T, Davis R: **The effect of eugenol-containing and eugenol-free temporary cements on microleakage in resin bonded restorations.** *Oper Dent* 1992, 17:175–180.

16. Barghi N, Knight GT, Berry TG: **Comparing two methods of moisture control in bonding to enamel: a clinical study.** *Oper Dent* 1991, 16:130–135.

17. Gwinnett AJ: **Effect of cavity disinfection on bond strength to dentin.** *J Esthet Dent* 1992, 4(suppl):11–13.

18. Nakabayashi N, Ashizawa M, Nakamura M: **Identification of a resin-dentin hybrid layer in vital human dentin created in vivo: durable bonding to vital dentin.** *Quintessence Int* 1992, 23:135–141.

19. Suh BI, Cincione FA: **All-Bond 2: the fourth generation bonding system.** *Esthet Dent Update* 1992, 3:61–66.

20. Nakabayashi N, Nakamura M, Yasuda N: **Hybrid layer as a dentin-bonding mechanism.** *J Esthet Dent* 1991, 4:133–138.

21. Kanca J: **Resin bonding to wet substrate: 1. Bonding to dentin.** *Quintessence Int* 1992, 23:39–41.
•• Benchmark study that shows definitively that etching dentin is desirable for increased bond strength and that no pulpal harm results from it.

22. O'Neal SJ, Miracle RL, Leinfelder KF: **Clinical evaluation of interfacial gaps for esthetic inlays.** *J Am Dent Assoc* 1993, 124:48–54.

William G. Dickerson, DDS, 4011 Meadows Lane, Las Vegas, NV 89107, USA.

Porcelain veneer adhesion systems

Frederick W. Costello, DDS

Ormond Beach, Florida, USA

The outstanding bonds achieved by composite resin luting systems to etched enamel and to etched and silanated porcelain are well documented. These bond strengths, in concert with the excellent and ever-improving dentin bonding systems, encourage the use of porcelain veneers in a continually expanding range of clinical situations and ensure predictable results. Clinicians desiring to offer their patients ultimate cosmetics in conjunction with optimal, conservative restorative techniques will need to monitor scientific and clinical results obtained by leaders in the field of adhesive dentistry and continually update their technique. This review brings the clinician up to date on current research and gives the clinician an understanding of the components of today's adhesive systems technology.

The state of the art of dentistry practice today has advanced far beyond the practice of 1980, and it will be considered primitive in the year 2010. The ever-expanding technology of adhesive dentistry is creating new solutions to traditional problems and is opening our minds to new benefits we can offer our patients. The outstanding predictability in the use of porcelain veneers is a direct result of the advancements in adhesive systems (Table 1).

Table 1. Uses of porcelain veneers
Current uses
Change teeth color from unacceptable or normal to beautiful
Alter the shape or size of teeth
Widen the arch and thus broaden the smile
Restore caries-damaged teeth or carious discoloration
Restore cracked and age-worn teeth
Close diastemata
Restore teeth worn and fractured from parafunctional habits
Mask tetracycline discoloration, fluorosis, other opacities and hypoplastic defects
Improve alignment of teeth (including postorthodontic relapse)
Correct horizontal plane and midline
Potential uses with newer bonding and adhesive systems
Replace missing teeth
Splint periodontally compromised teeth
Restore and improve functional pathways of occlusion

Humble beginnings

Porcelain veneers have been used in one form or another since 1937, when they were retained with denture adhesive; later, they were cemented with acrylic resin [1••]. Beginning in 1983, when Simonsen and Calamia [2] described improved retention by etching porcelain with 7.5% hydrofluoric acid, and 1984, when the same authors reported on the effect of coupling agents on the bond strength of porcelain [3], porcelain veneers have become predictable when bonded to etched enamel. Sorenson et al.'s [4] 1990 report that microleakage was all but eliminated when etching and silanating of the porcelain were combined [4] and Blair et al.'s [5•] 1993 study that showed use of a dentin bonding agent with a composite resin cement will reduce microleakage at the dentin-cementum margin continued the advancement of this exciting technique.

In a well-documented 5-year clinical study by Dunne and Millar [1••], 83% of 315 porcelain labial veneers fitted in 96 patients between 1986 and 1991 were deemed satisfactory at recall. Minimal problem and failure rates were associated with veneers placed on existing restorations, where tooth surface loss had occurred prior to treatment (although teeth with more than 50% of enamel and tooth structure loss were excluded), and where inappropriate luting agents were employed. Our adhesion materials and techniques are constantly improving, which can only increase the success rates published in future studies (Fig. 1).

Today's systems

The high bond strength of porcelain to enamel appears to be a critical factor in the excellent clini-

58   Cosmetic dentistry

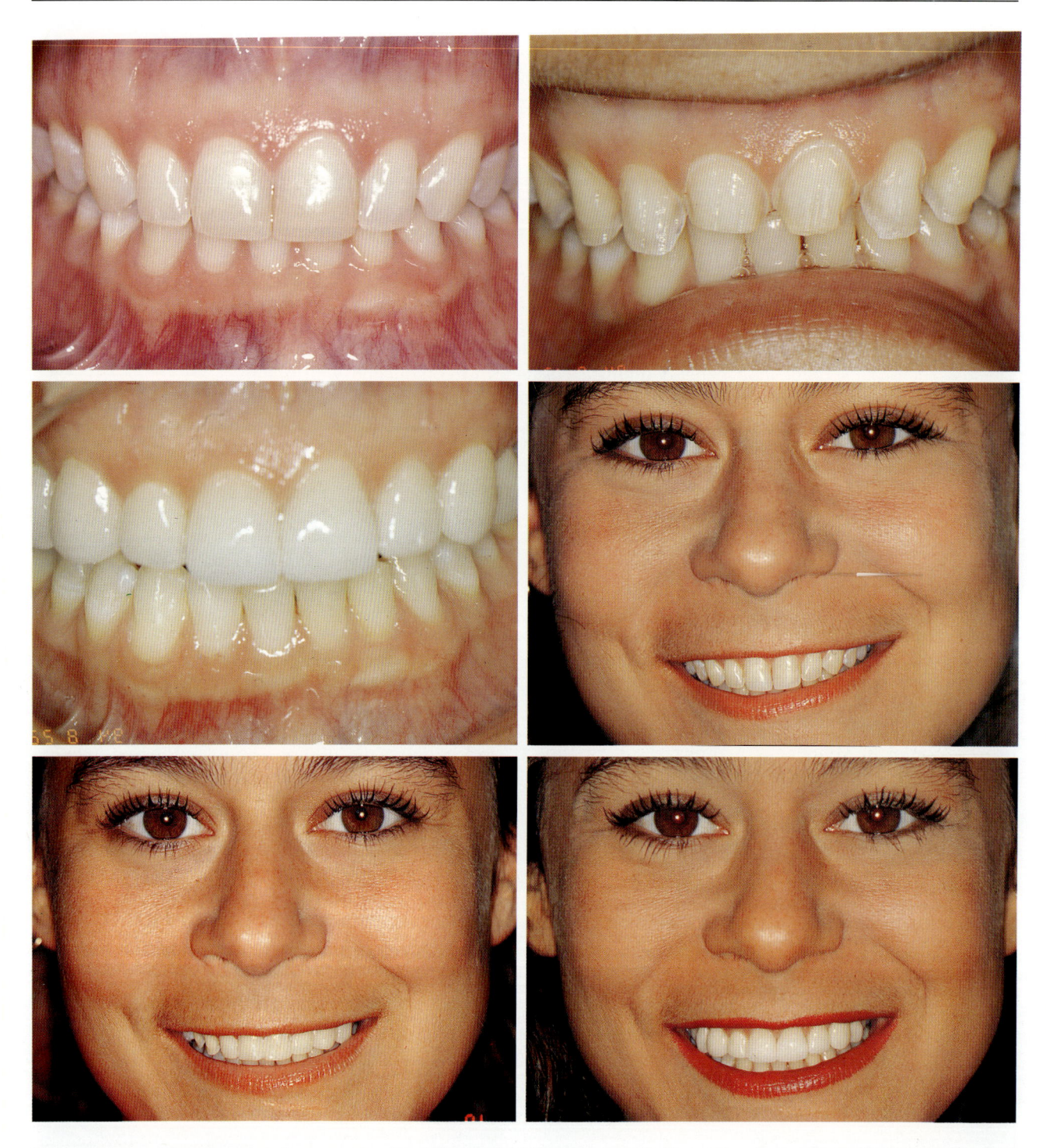

Fig. 1. A 27-year-old woman wanted to correct her thin "chicken teeth." She also wanted whiter teeth and a broader smile. Veneers were used to widen teeth, and bulking out of the bicuspids gave a fuller, broader smile. **Top left,** Anterior view before the procedure. Note discolored direct bonding on central incisors. **Top right,** Preparation of teeth 5 to 12. All composite resin was removed from teeth 8 and 9. **Center left,** After application of porcelain veneers, shade A-1, seated with Mirage Light Catalyst and B-1 base (Chameleon Dental Products, Kansas City, KS). **Center right,** Full facial view before the procedure. **Bottom left,** Temporary veneers were placed on teeth 5 to 10 and dentin primer on teeth 11 and 12, so that patient could see how a broader smile would look. **Bottom right,** After the procedure.

cal success achieved with bonding of porcelain veneers. In a study by Barkmeier *et al.* [6••], the bond strength of porcelain to enamel was significantly higher than the bond strength to dentin. Although the obtained porcelain bond strengths to dentin were comparatively higher than many previously reported values for composite resin to dentin using various adhesive systems, enamel bond strengths were clearly superior when compared with those of dentin. The results indicated that clinical preparations should be limited to enamel whenever possible, but that the newer generation of adhesive systems shows excellent potential for bonding to dentin (Tables 2 and 3). We can expect the dentin bonding measurements to be even higher with wet bonding, which was not used in this study.

Bleaching and bonding are often combined. It has been reported that it is best to wait 1 week after bleaching before bonding [7,8]. If bonding must be done immediately after bleaching, Barghi and Godwin [9] described a successful technique using a water displacement solution (alcohol or acetone) and a dentin bonding agent that contains acetone.

The components of adhesion systems

Etched porcelain veneer
There was no significant difference in the mean flexural strengths between the etched and nonetched porcelains and no significant difference between the different etching times for either porcelain or castable glass ceramics; it therefore appears that chemical etching can improve the retention of ceramic laminate veneers without significant loss of strength [10•,11•].

Silane coupler
Silane treatment of the etched porcelain resulted in a significantly greater shear strength when compared with the samples that were merely etched. Silane-treated bonds of porcelain to composite resin were stronger than the bonds of enamel to composite resin. Thermocycling did not significantly diminish the shear bond strength for the enamel or silane-treated porcelain to composite resin samples [12•].

Unfilled resin adhesive
It is not advisable to cure the unfilled resin adhesive prior to luting the veneer in place, because the thickness of the adhesive film may compromise the fit of the veneer. Use of a dual-cure unfilled resin adhesive significantly reduces the working time of some dual-cure composite resin luting cements. The chemical component of the polymerization of a dual-cure luting composite may be accelerated if excess activator is present in the dual cure unfilled resin adhesive, such as when Bondlite (Kerr Manufacturing Co., Romulus, MI) is used with Porcelite Dual Cure (Kerr Manufacturing Co.) [13]. The PreBond in the All-Bond 2 System (Bisco, Itasca, IL) answers this potential problem by slowing down the polymerization process. The ScotchBond Multi-Purpose Plus system (3M Dental Products, St. Paul, MN) addresses this situation by using the catalyst without the adhesive, which delays polymerization until the catalyst comes in contact with the dual-cure luting composite resin (Table 4).

Table 2. Criteria for the final generation of dentin bonding agents

Bond strength to cementum, dentin, and enamel equal to cohesive bond of tooth structure

Total seal of dentin tubules	Gap-free bond	No microleakage
Biologic compatibility	Palliative to pulp	Antibacterial
Bondability to moist or dry surfaces	No polymerization shrinkage	Clinically proven
Universal composite-porcelain-metal compatibility	Instant bond	Fluoride release
Toothlike coefficient of expansion and contraction	Freedom from hydrolysis	Low film thickness
Self, dual, or photo-initiated cure	Ease of handling	Unlimited shelf life
Stimulation of reparative dentin bridge for predictable direct and indirect pulp capping		Low cost

Bonding to and subsequent remineralization of carious dentin
No self-discoloration (or discoloration of other materials) over time or under ultraviolet light rays
Bonding with or without tooth mechanical or chemical preparation

Table 3. Criteria for the ideal composite resin luting agent

Bond strength to dentin enamel primer and unfilled resin adhesive and to etched, silanated porcelain and metal (via unfilled resin adhesive) exceeds bond strength of dentin enamel primer and unfilled resin to tooth

Biologic compatibility	Antibacterial	Clinically proven
No polymerization shrinkage	Low film thickness	No microleakage
Toothlike coefficient of expansion and contraction	Freedom from hydrolysis	No postoperative sensitivity
No oxygen-inhibited zone	Plaque will not adhere	Fluoride release
Variable opacity, translucency	Variable consistency	Variable setting time
No discoloration	Shade consistency	Surface will not stain
Easily tintable before or after set	Ease of handling	Easy removal of excess
Self, dual, or photo-initiated infinite cure	Unlimited shelf life	Low cost

Table 4. Popular adhesive bonding systems

Optibond (Kerr Manufacturing Co., Romulus, MI)
  Kit includes light-cure prime, light-cure resin adhesive, dual-cure resin adhesive (activator and paste), applicators
ScotchBond Multi-Purpose Adhesive System (3M Dental Products, St. Paul, MN)
  Kit includes etchant, primer, adhesive
ScotchBond Multi-Purpose Plus Adhesive System (3M Dental Products)
  Kit includes Scothbond ceramic primer, etchant, activator, primer, and adhesive and catalyst
All-Bond 2 (Bisco, Itasca, IL)
  Kit includes primers A and B, dentin and enamel bonding resin, prebond, etchant
Adhesive by Choice/Enhanced (Chameleon Dental Products, Kansas City, KS)
  Kit includes nitric acid conditioner, H_3PO_4, primer parts A, B, and C (for metal bonding), unfilled resin base and catalyst, acidulated phosphofluoride, silane
Tenure (Den-Mat Corp., Santa Maria, CA)
  Kit includes dentin conditioner, primer A and B, Visar seal (unfilled adhesive resin); Tenure S is an update to the Visar seal
Permagen (Ultradent Products, Salt Lake City, UT)
  Kit includes primer A and B, light-cured bonding resin, 35% and 10% etch, porcelain etch
PowerBond (Cosmedent, Chicago, IL)
  Kit includes dentin conditioner, primer A and B, light-cure resin (3A), dual-cure resin catalyst (3B)
ProBOND Adhesive System (Caulk Co., Milford, DE)
  Kit includes primer, adhesive

Composite resin luting agents

The clinician may choose a light-cure or a dual-cure system for porcelain veneers. According to Christensen [14•], light-cure materials are most popular for porcelain veneers because of the occasional need to remove the veneer before curing and the slight color change in some dual-cure cements over a period of service. I have found that with proper try-in techniques, the need to remove a veneer before curing is all but eliminated. Clinicians who usually prefer light-cure may revert to dual-cure materials when there has been more than minimal tooth preparation, or where the veneer is thicker than usual (eg, lingually inclined teeth) or more opaque than usual to mask underlying tooth discoloration (Figs. 1 and 2).

Dual-cure composite resin cements combine the autocuring components (ie, amine and peroxide accelerators) of the self-cure resins with the photosensitizer (ie, camphorquinone) contained in the light-cure resins. Compared with self-curing composite resins, dual-cure composite resins contain a decreased concentration of autocuring accelerators, which reduces the potential for discoloration, but they do contain more autocuring accelerators and hence present a greater chance of discoloration than the light-cure composites. It is advisable to treat dual-cure materials as light-cure materials, because the manufacturers of some dual-cure materials stipulate that they do not reach their full hardness from self-curing for 24 hours; despite manufacturers' claims, there is no evidence that a substantial chemically induced polymerization of dual-cure resins occurs after light exposure is completed. For most resin systems tested, the cure observed 10 minutes postmix was almost equivalent to the cure after 24 hours [15•]. Higher levels of hardness were obtained with dual-cure resin cements (Table 5) [16•].

The output of the light source is a major component of any light-cure or dual-cure adhesion system. The degree of polymerization initiated by the curing light controls the esthetic quality and the clinical performance of the material. Maximum output of the light units may be significantly reduced by a variety of documented factors [17•]. Also, porcelain has been shown to absorb between 40% and 50% of the light so cure the luting composite resins under the porcelain veneers for longer than conventional composite materials in order to achieve full polymerization [18].

A strong correlation was found between film thickness and consistency which was supported by the temperature dependence of film thickness reported for the dual cure luting composites. Cooling of the material increased the consistency, resulting in a larger film thickness, whereas heating reduced the film thickness because of the lower consistency [19••].

Dentin bonding and primer

According to Jordan et al. [20••], the original dentin bond resins were introduced to the profession in the early 1980s, and although they were a step in the right direction, they had a bond strength of only 6 MPa and could not stand the polymerization contraction of the composite materials placed on them. The stress from polymerization contraction inevitably resulted in the formation of a gap at the resin-dentin interface that ultimately led to the failure of the restoration in the form of microleakage in association with recurrent caries, postoperative sensitivity, or both. These older-generation dentin bonding agents gave dentin bonding a bad name. All of the new generation of universal dentin bonding materials offer the potential of withstanding composite polymerization contraction shrinkage without gap formation. These new dentin systems bond extremely well to enamel, dentin, porcelain, and metallic surfaces, with bond strengths of 18 to 20 MPa, more closely approximating the strength of resin's bond to acid-etched enamel of 18 MPa, which is virtually indestructible and gap free [20••].

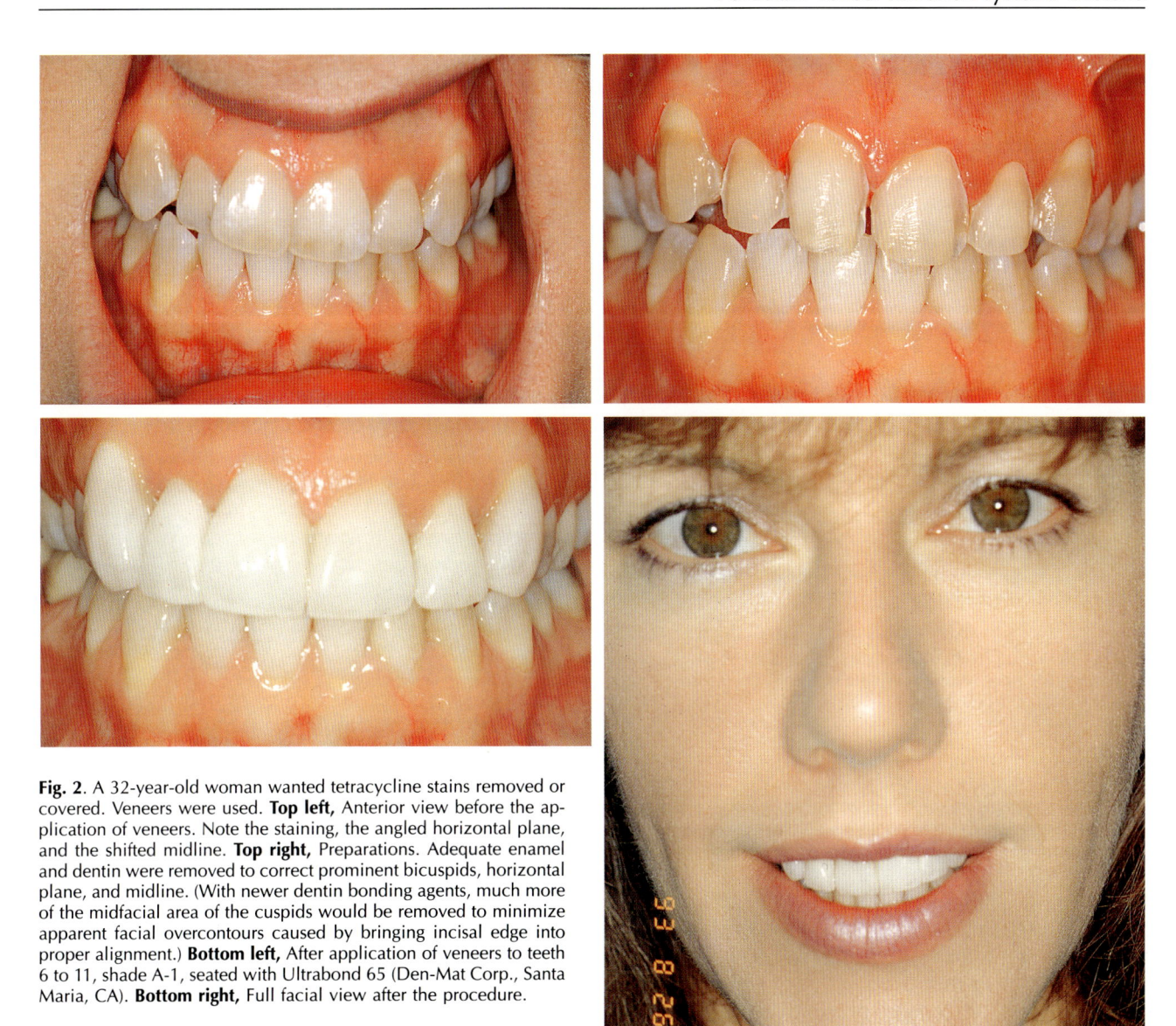

Fig. 2. A 32-year-old woman wanted tetracycline stains removed or covered. Veneers were used. **Top left,** Anterior view before the application of veneers. Note the staining, the angled horizontal plane, and the shifted midline. **Top right,** Preparations. Adequate enamel and dentin were removed to correct prominent bicuspids, horizontal plane, and midline. (With newer dentin bonding agents, much more of the midfacial area of the cuspids would be removed to minimize apparent facial overcontours caused by bringing incisal edge into proper alignment.) **Bottom left,** After application of veneers to teeth 6 to 11, shade A-1, seated with Ultrabond 65 (Den-Mat Corp., Santa Maria, CA). **Bottom right,** Full facial view after the procedure.

Here comes the obligatory description of the chemistry involved. The dentin primer (hydrophilic monomer) used in current "fourth-generation" dentin bonding wets the dentin surface and cohesively infiltrates the etched vital intratubular dentin, forming resin tags and helping to form the hybridized zone (resin-impregnated layer) that facilitates the bond between the dentin and the composite resin [21•]. This process minimizes patient postoperative hypersensitivity, prevents future microleakage through the dentin-resin–hybridized interface, and is totally biocompatible to the pulp [22•].

The effect of the dentin bonding agents on shear bond strength to enamel has been questioned. Dickerson [23•] studied Optibond (Kerr Manufacturing Co.) and showed that if the proper protocol is followed, bond strengths to enamel were not diminished. He believed that perhaps other studies showing a decreased enamel bond had failed to dry the dentin primer adequately before placing the enamel bonding resin, and he believed that a residue of primer left on the surface would interfere with the bond strength [23•]. Current techniques include instructions to make sure the primer is dry and shiny before applying the adhesive resin.

The simple, no-mix dentin bonding systems with primers and one-component, light-cure, unfilled bonding resins are typically designed to be used with direct restorations. When using one-component systems as ScotchBond MP (3M Dental Products), Optibond (using a no-mix, light-cure adhesive resin), and Aelite Bond (Bisco) for porcelain veneers, the thickness of the primers or resin layers which typically require light curing prior to restoration placement may compromise the fit of the veneer.

Table 5. Popular composite resin luting agents

Porcelite (Kerr Manufacturing Co., Romulus, MI)
  Kit includes porcelain primer, etchant, Bondlite, 4 shades of
    base (2 additional shades are available, including an opaquer)
Porcelite Dual Cure (Kerr Manufacturing Co.)
  Kit includes procelain primer, Bondlite, 4 shades of base
    (2 additional shades are available, including an opaquer)
Indirect Porcelain Dentist Bonding Kit (3M Dental Products,
  St. Paul, MN)
  Kit contains Scotchprime ceramic primer (silane), 7 light-cure
    A shades (including clear), 7 catalyst B shades (including clear)
    for dual cure that can also be used for try-in
Ultrabond (Den-Mat Corp., Santa Maria, CA)
  Various formulations are available
Mirage FLC Plus (Chameleon Dental Products, Kansas City, KS)
  Kit includes 5 Vita shades of base (no opaque shades), 2 shades
    of self-cure catalyst, A and B primers from the ABC enhanced kit,
    silane
EnForce (Caulk Co., Milford, DE)
  Kit includes tooth conditioner, ProBOND primer, ProBOND adhesive,
    5 base shades, blending paste (makes base light-cure), catalyst
    (makes base self-cure)
Insure and Insure Lite (Cosmedent, Chicago, IL)
  Kit contains cements and Simulcure, color modifiers, silane, Etch
    Protect, PorcelEtch, glycerin
Choice (Bisco, Itasca, IL)
  Kit contains etchant, procelain primer, dental adhesive, 4 shades
    of cement (10 are available), dual-cure catalyst, Biscolor (8 shades),
    try-in pastes (water soluble or regular)
Variolink Resin Luting System (Ivoclar-Vivadent, Amherst, NY)
  Kit includes 2 catalyst viscosities (thick and thin), continuous
    fluoride release, high radiopacity, high translucency, light-
    or dual-cured, and 3 base shades that correspond with cured try-in
    pastes (base used without catalyst is light-cured only);
    professional set includes everything needed for adhesive luting

Dual-cure systems such as Tenure (Den-Mat Corp., Santa Maria, CA), All-Bond 2, Optibond (using their two component dual cure adhesive resin), and Permagen (Ultradent Products, Salt Lake City, UT) typically require the mixing of primers or bonding resins and thus are not as easy to use and typically take more time. They are designed so they may be used with indirect restorations.

When a dentin bonding agent is used in conjunction with luting materials, it is essential that the dentin bonding agent is of low film thickness, so that the fit of the veneer is not prejudiced, especially if you light cure the resin prior to placing the indirect restoration, as some manufacturers recommend. *Reality* recommends against curing bonding resins prior to luting indirect restorations [24]. I agree.

3M has recently announced the development of ScotchBond Multi-Purpose Plus, which adds an activator and catalyst to their system, thus improving the flexibility to an already outstanding system by allowing its use in self-cure and dual-cure applications, as well as light cure. It surely will not be long before other manufacturers follow suit and introduce adhesion systems with variable component combinations for use in all situations.

Because discoloration of aging primers indicates a potential for a reduced bond strength, and the chemistry is advancing so rapidly, it is not wise to buy dentin bonding systems in bulk. Use fresh material and pay close attention to expiration dates [25].

Etched enamel, dentin, and cementum

At the 1994 American Academy of Cosmetic Dentistry meeting in Phoenix, Kanca [26] went beyond discussing the total etch technique, discovery of the hybrid layer formation, and development of the wet technique, which have given us reliable bonding agents for adhesion to dentin, and discussed pulp capping via etching and use of dentin bonding agents. If the current research has passed beyond questioning the efficacy of total etch dentin bonding and gone on to the benefits versus potential drawbacks of pulp capping by etching and dentin bonding, it seems time to accept dentin bonding as here to stay. As long as the etched dentin surface, also called the demineralized zone, is properly sealed, the action of the etchant will not harm the pulp, provided the etched surface is sealed quickly to prevent bacterial contamination.

Porcelain veneers versus composite resin veneers or crowns

Lacy *et al.* [27] and Tam and McComb [28] reported no microleakage of veneers bonded to etched enamel, limited microleakage on the resin-dentin interface, and higher microleakage for composite veneers over porcelain veneers due to their higher coefficients of thermal expansion.

When teeth were struck on the middle labial surface by a pendulum impact device, porcelain veneers were remarkably resistant to fracture; fractures occurred only at the site of impact and the veneers remained cemented. Patterns of fracture were similar to those for intact, unrestored teeth. Porcelain veneers and full gold crowns stiffened teeth, leaking to more root fractures than porcelain crowns. Dicor crowns (Dentsply International, York, PA) were less fracture-resistant than the other restorations tested [29•].

Adhesive temporization

I have come to believe that when you are doing a cosmetic procedure, you should never send patients away from your office looking worse than they did when they walked in. The benefits of temporization far outweigh the time of fabrication and time and potential frustration associated with removal. You must remove all of the composite resin used in temporization. I have found the following method of temporization best achieves a balance between retention and easy removal: use a 3-mm diameter spot of etch in the center of the tooth, coat the teeth with a dentin bonding agent for sensitivity protection (no adhesive resin), and then sculpt the old composite resin as a blueprint for the final veneers and as a one-piece cosmetic temporary (Figs. 1, 3, and 4).

Shading

Two shade guides of the same origin can present completely different fluorescence. The cementing medium can affect the fluorescence of a ceramic prosthesis [30]. Because of metamerism, color-matched objects under one illuminant will appear unmatched under a different illuminant. Color changes occurring in the thin layers of dual-cure composite resin cements may not be clinically significant; this potential color change would not be as important in cases of multiple veneers [31•].

How can we ever get the shade right? Many excellent resin tint kits are available that are compatible with any luting composite resin system. Resin tints can make significant shade changes if the porcelain veneer is thin and translucent. Therefore, when in doubt about a shade, go light, and after determining the proper shade with the try-in pastes, tint the luting composite resin to the proper shade. It is the discrepancy between the surface reflection and the internal reflection that provides the illusion of transparency, such that if the internal reflection is greater than the surface reflection, you will have an opaque material; if the internal reflection is less than the surface reflection you will have a transparent material. Chpindel and Cristou [32••] described a double-layer porcelain veneer technique that allows the discrepancy between the surface porcelain's increased translucent reflection and the internal porcelain's diminished translucency reflec-

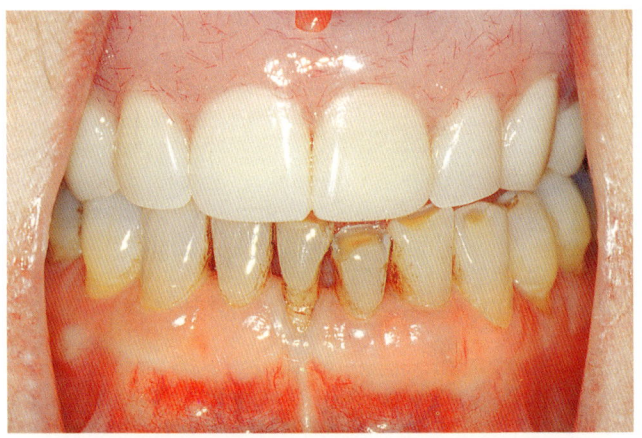

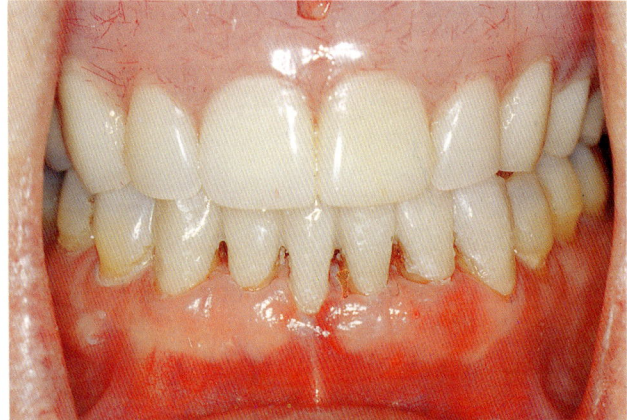

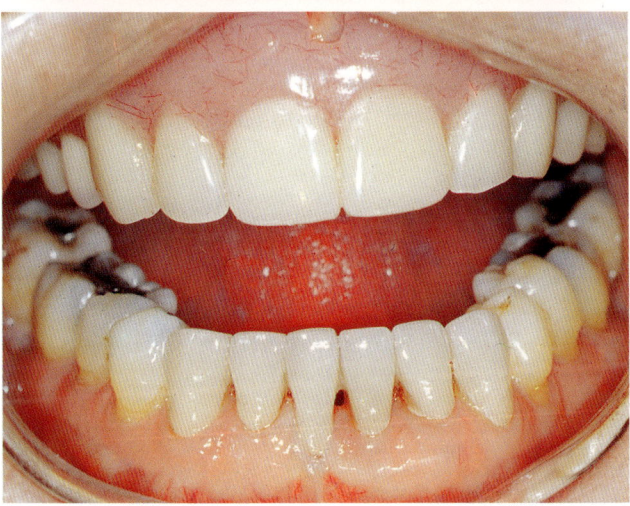

Fig. 3. A 70-year-old woman wanted her teeth to look less "worn out." Porcelain veneers were used. **Upper left,** Before the procedure. **Upper right,** Temporary veneers. **Bottom,** After application of porcelain veneers to teeth 22 to 27, shade A-3, seated with 3M Indirect Porcelain Dentist Bonding Kit Warm Medium Opacity (3M Dental Products, St. Paul, MN).

tion to give the illusion of transparency, which compared very favorably with the shade of natural teeth.

Cementation

Use water (when not evaluating shade considerations) or a try-in paste to check contacts, seating, and shade; tint the try-in paste as necessary. Water soluble try-in pastes are available with some composite resin systems, whereas other systems are compatible with the resin cements and do not have to be fully cleaned out if the shade is acceptable. I have found that selection of a try-in paste that is easy to use and clean out will likely influence you to use it routinely. It will save you time. Etch the enamel, dentin, cementum with 30% to 40% phosphoric acid for 15 to 20 seconds [33•], rinse, and leave slightly moist; apply 2% chlorhexidine to damp dentin [34], dry the surface slightly, leaving the surface moist, and then apply dentin primer, and cure if so directed. Clean the veneer as directed, briefly re-etch with hydrofluoric acid, rinse, dry, and silanate [12•]. Decide on light- or dual-cure resin, coat the tooth (which should be shiny and dry), and veneer with unfilled bonding resin just prior to adding the composite resin luting agent.

I routinely use ScotchBond Multi-Purpose Primer because it seems to be the simplest of the high-bond dentin primers: no mix, one coat, dry for 5 seconds, and immediately (with no waiting or light-curing) coat with an unfilled resin adhesive. If you are using a light-cure composite resin luting agent, use a light-cure unfilled resin such as ScotchBond Multi-Purpose Adhesive. Because I prefer the extra security afforded with dual cure, I have been using a dual-cure unfilled resin such as Bondlite, but I am also excited about the new ScotchBond Multi-Purpose Plus system. I have tried many composite resin luting agents, but among the dual cures, Porcelite Dual Cure is my favorite, primarily because my assistants like its handling properties, and I do like to keep them happy. I also like the Vita (Vita Zahnfabrik, Bad Säckingen, FRG) shades in the Mirage FLC Plus (Chameleon Dental Products, Kansas City, KS) for light-cure seating of thin, relatively translucent single veneers, when I am most concerned about the potential for color degradation over time and least concerned about depth of cure.

The presence of oxygen prevents polymerizing of the surface layer of composite resin materials, and resin cements may be affected unless protected by a matrix or other means, *eg*, the application of a glycerin gel, such as De-Ox (Ultradent Products, Salt Lake City, UT), to the exposed resin cement surface to prevent the formation of the oxygen-inhibited layer.

The future of adhesion

To date, the main limitation of adhesive restorations has been the insufficient dentinal bonding in clinical situations that presented us with thin gingival enamel margins. Adhesive fractures on dentin or near the cementoenamel junction will lead to marginal or internal leakage, which is responsible for dentinal pain, recurrent caries, and injuries to the pulp [35•]. Although microleakage does not directly correlate with clinical failure, it has been associated with postoperative sensitivity, recurrent caries, marginal staining, and pulpal pathosis [5•].

Freedman [36] said that ease, speed, and the range of utilization in a variety of situations are important, but he rarely asked questions that would play an important role in the dentist's choice of bonding system; bond strengths are not a great differentiating factor. It is comforting to know that the issue is not whether the material will work, but which material is the easiest to work with.

In response to the improvements in dentin bonding, leading clinicians are stretching the envelope [37,38•,39•,40–44]. We are using porcelain veneers on teeth with extensive previous enamel destruction and subsequent restoration because we can reliably bond to dentin where previously full coverage would have been indicated (Fig. 2). At the 1994 American Academy of Cosmetic Dentistry meeting in Phoenix, Barghi (Unpublished lecture) talked about "taco shell" veneers (*ie*, those covering the facial and lingual surfaces while leav-

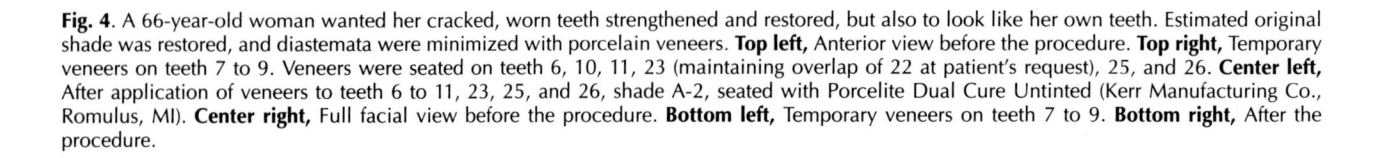

Fig. 4. A 66-year-old woman wanted her cracked, worn teeth strengthened and restored, but also to look like her own teeth. Estimated original shade was restored, and diastemata were minimized with porcelain veneers. **Top left,** Anterior view before the procedure. **Top right,** Temporary veneers on teeth 7 to 9. Veneers were seated on teeth 6, 10, 11, 23 (maintaining overlap of 22 at patient's request), 25, and 26. **Center left,** After application of veneers to teeth 6 to 11, 23, 25, and 26, shade A-2, seated with Porcelite Dual Cure Untinted (Kerr Manufacturing Co., Romulus, MI). **Center right,** Full facial view before the procedure. **Bottom left,** Temporary veneers on teeth 7 to 9. **Bottom right,** After the procedure.

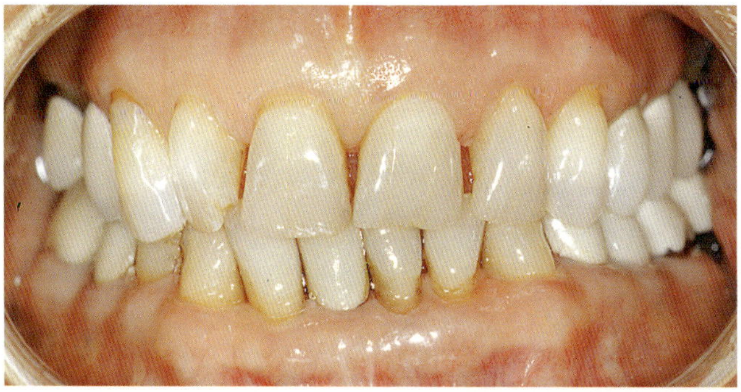

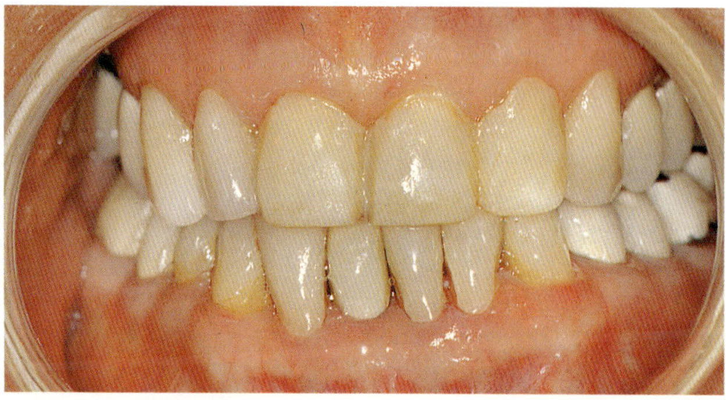

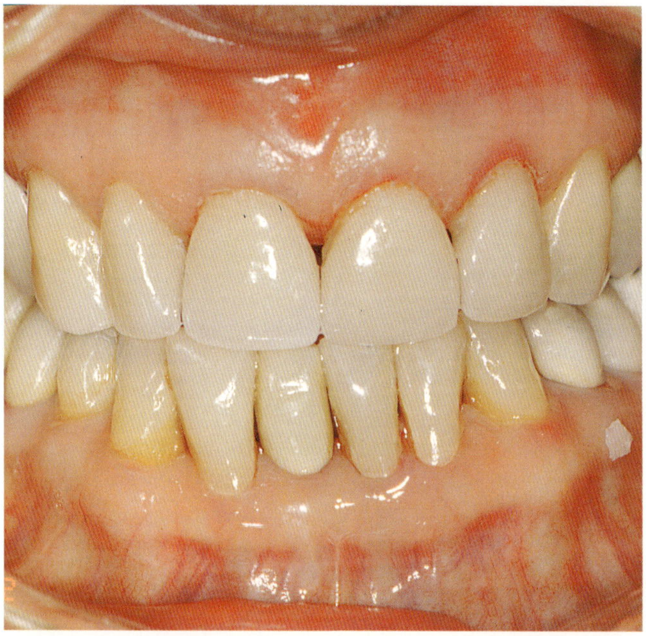

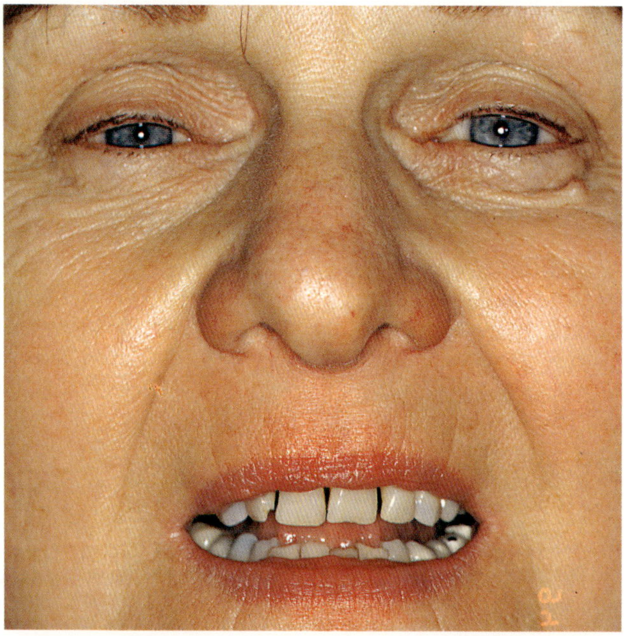

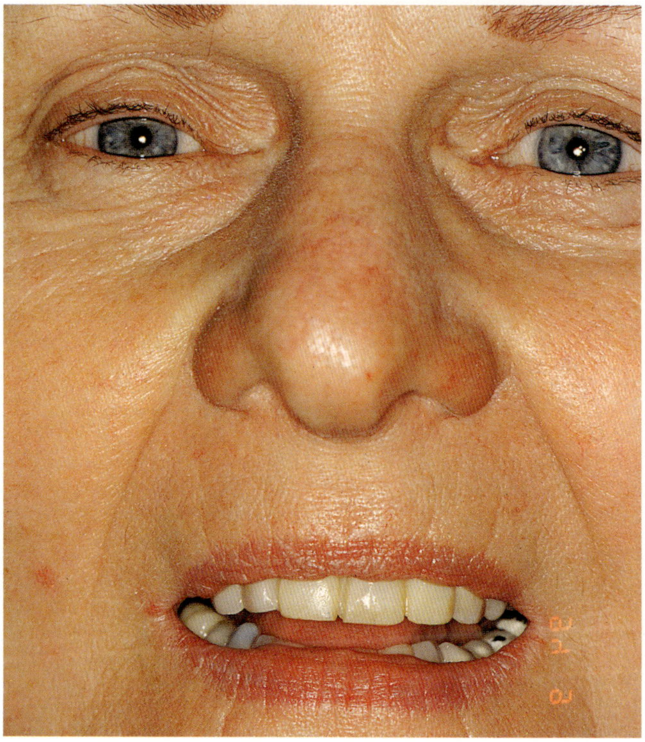

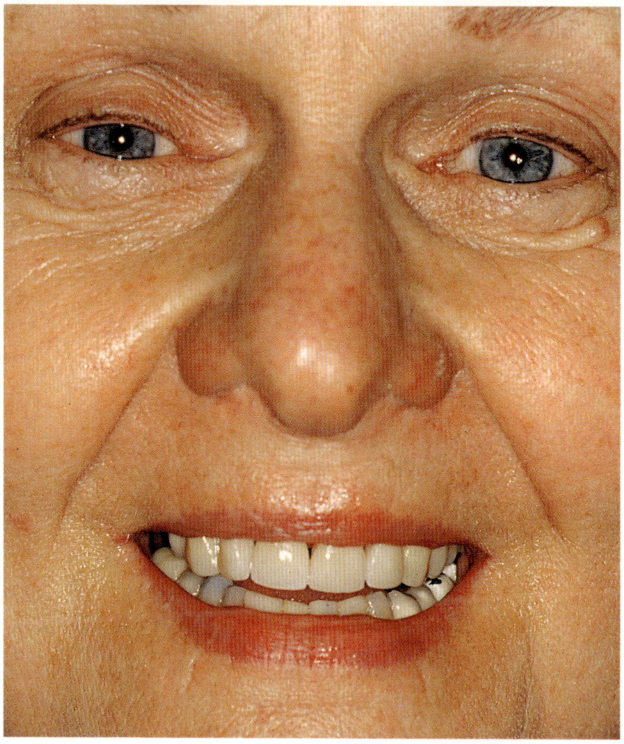

ing proximal surfaces intact), incisal tip veneers to restore lost incisal edges and cingulum veneers in maxillary cuspids when opposed by mandibular porcelain. Denissen *et al.* [45••] reported an encouraging 75% success rate after 5 years with 12 porcelain veneer fixed partial dentures; can the acceptance horizon for this technique be far removed? Will we be able to bond off-the-shelf porcelain facings sized only for width and incisal length with no concern for marginal fit? Will advanced adhesive systems allow us to do away with all indirect restorations, once the handling, cosmetic, and physical properties of direct adhesive restorative materials rival those of indirect composite resins, porcelain, and gold?

Conclusions

Resin luting agents have several advantages: they can be bonded to enamel, dentin, and etched porcelain, reportedly strengthening the restoration. Ceramic crowns bonded with a dual polymerizing resin cement have been shown to have twice the load resistance of crowns luted with zinc phosphate cement. Resin-bonded porcelain crowns and porcelain veneers have been shown to be as fracture resistant as unprepared teeth. The resin to porcelain bond may exceed the cohesive strength of the resin cement. The cosmetics of porcelain veneers is unsurpassed.

We clinicians are constantly challenged to balance our conservative natures and the prudence of waiting until a technique is tried, tested, and true with our desire to be on the "cutting edge." Patients love the cosmetic results obtained with porcelain veneers. The current techniques are simple when you follow the directions for each material, and we have well documented clinical studies showing excellent results using older materials that are inferior to those available today. There is no reason to wait. Welcome to adhesive dentistry!

References and recommended reading

Papers of particular interest, published within the annual period of review, have been highlighted as:
- Of special interest
- •• Of outstanding interest

1. Dunne SM, Millar BJ: **A longitudinal study of the clin-**
•• **ical performance of porcelain veneers.** *Br Dent J* 1993, 175:317–321.
Of 315 porcelain labial veneers fitted in 96 patients between 1986 and 1991, 83% were deemed satisfactory. Increased problem and failure rates were associated with veneers placed on existing restorations, where tooth surface loss had occurred prior to treatment (although teeth with greater than 50% of enamel and tooth structure loss were excluded) and where inappropriate luting agents were employed.

2. Simonsen RJ, Calamia JR: **Tensile bond strength of etched porcelain** [abstract]. *J Dent Res* 1983, 62(special issue):abstract 1154.

3. Calamia JR, Simonsen RJ: **The effect of coupling agents on bond strength of etched porcelain.** *J Dent Res* 1984, 63:179.

4. Sorenson JA, Kang SK, Avera SA: **Microleakage of composite to various porcelain surface treatments** [abstract]. *J Dent Res* 1990, 69:359.

5. Blair KF, Koeppen RG, Schwartz RS, Davis RD: **Microleak-**
• **age associated with resin composite-cemented, cast glass ceramic restoration.** *Int J Prosthodont* 1993, 6:579–584.
A dentin bonding agent with a resin cement reduced microleakage at the dentin-cementum margin.

6. Barkmeier WW, Menis DL, Barnes DM: **Bond strength of a**
•• **veneering porcelain using newer generation adhesive systems.** *Pract Periodontics Aesthet Dent* 1994, 5:50–55.
The results of this study indicated that clinical preparations should be limited to enamel when possible, but that the newer-generation adhesive systems show excellent potential for bonding to dentin. We can expect these dentin bonding measurements to be even higher with wet bonding, which was not used in this study.

7. Haywood VB, Williams HA: **Status and restorative options for dentist-prescribed home-applied bleaching.** *Esthet Dent Update* 1994, 5:65.

8. Tiley KC, Torneck CD, Ruse ND: **The effect of carbamide-peroxide gel on the shear bond strength of a microfil resin to bovine enamel.** *J Dent Res* 1992, 71:20–24.

9. Barghi N, Godwin JM: **Reducing the adverse effect of bleaching on composite-enamel bond.** *J Esthet Dent* 1994, 6:157–161.

10. Yen T, Blackman RB, Baez RJ: **Effect of acid etching on the**
• **flexural strength of a feldspathic porcelain and a castable glass ceramic.** *J Prosthet Dent* 1993, 70:224–233.
Chemical etching can improve the retention of ceramic laminate veneers without significant loss of strength.

11. Wolf DM, Powers JM, O'Keefe KL: **Bond strength of com-**
• **posite to etched and sandblasted porcelain.** *Am J Dent* 1993, 6:155–158.
High *in vitro* bond strengths for bonding of porcelain veneers with a composite resin can be obtained by etching with Ceram-Etch gel (Gresco Products, Stafford, TX) for 2.5 minutes or blasting with 48 μm aluminum oxide.

12. Stacey GD: **A shear stress analysis of the bonding of porce-**
• **lain veneers to enamel.** *J Prosthet Dent* 1993, 70:395–402.
Silane treatment of the etched porcelain produced a significantly greater shear strength to the merely etched samples. Silane-treated porcelain–composite resin bonds were stronger than the enamel–composite resin bonds. Thermocycling did not significantly diminish the shear bond strength of the enamel or silane-treated porcelain to composite resin samples.

13. Shortall AD, Baylis RL, Fisher SE, Harrington E: **Operating variables affecting the working time of a dual-cure composite luting cement.** *Eur J Prosthodont Restor Dent* 1993, 1:185–188.

14. Christensen GJ: **The rise of resin for cementing restora-**
• **tions.** *J Am Dent Assoc* 1993, 124:104–105.

Light-cure materials are most popular for porcelain veneers because of the occasional need to remove the veneer before curing, and the slight color change in some dual-cure cements over a period of service.

15. Rueggeberg FA, Caughman WF: **The influence of light exposure on polymerization of dual-cure resin cements.** *Oper Dent* 1993, **18**:48–55.

Despite manufacturers' claims, there is no evidence for a substantial, chemically induced polymerization of dual-cure resins occurring after light exposure is completed. For most resin systems tested, the cure observed 10 minutes postmix was almost equivalent to the cure after 24 hours.

16. Cardash HS, Baharav H, Pilo R, Ben-Amar A: **The effect of porcelain color on the hardness of luting composite resin cement.** *J Prosthet Dent* 1993, **69**:620–623.

Higher levels of hardness were obtained with dual-cure resin cements.

17. Barghi N, Berry T, Hatton C: **Evaluating intensity output of curing lights in private dental offices.** *J Am Dent Assoc* 1994, **125**:992–996.

The degree of polymerization initiated by the curing light controls the esthetic quality and the clinical performance of the material. Maximum output of the light units may be significantly reduced by a variety of documented factors.

18. Burke FJT, McCaughey AD: **Resin luting materials: the current status.** *Dent Update* 1993, **20**:109–115.

19. Van Meerbeek B, Inokoshi S, Davidson CL, De Gee AJ, Landrechts P, Bralm M, Vaherle G: **Dual cure luting composites. Part II: clinically related properties.** *J Oral Rehabil* 1994, **21**:57–66.

Thirteen dual-cure luting composites were compared for film thickness, consistency, and working time. A strong correlation was found between film thickness and consistency, which was supported by the temperature dependence of film thickness of dual-cure luting composites. Cooling of the material increased the consistency, resulting in a larger film thickness, whereas heating reduced the film thickness because of the lower consistency.

20. Jordan RE, Suzuki M, Davidson DF: **Clinical evaluation of a universal dentin bonding resin: preserving dentition through new materials.** *J Am Dent Assoc* 1993, **124**:71–76.

The new-generation universal dentin bonding materials all offer the potential of withstanding composite polymerization contraction without gap formation. These systems bond extremely well to enamel, dentin, porcelain, and metallic surfaces with dentin bond strengths of 18 to 20 MPa, which more closely approximate the strength of resin's bond to acid-etched enamel of 18 MPa, which is virtually indestructible and gap-free.

21. Ward DH: **Dentin bonding.** *Esthet Dent Update* 1994, **5**:98.

The dentin primer (hydrophilic monomer) used in current fourth-generation dentin bonding agents wets the dentin surface, cohesively infiltrates the etched vital intratubular dentin, and forms resin tags, which helps form the hybridized zone (*ie*, resin-impregnated layer) that facilitates the bond between the dentin and the composite resin when collagen fibrils entangle with polymer chains, resulting in increased bond strengths.

22. Cox CF, Suzuki S: **Re-evaluating pulp protection: calcium hydroxide liners vs. cohesive hybridization.** *J Am Dent Assoc* 1994, **125**:831.

These adhesive dentin primers and dentin bonding systems prevent postoperative hypersensitivity and microleakage through the dentin resin-hybridized interface. They are a rapid and cost-productive means of ensuring routine structural reinforcement of the underlying remaining dentin while being totally biocompatible to the pulp.

23. Dickerson WG: **The effect of a dentin primer on enamel bond strength.** *Esthet Dent Update* 1994, **5**:63.

If the proper protocol is followed, bond strengths to enamel with Optibond are not diminished.

24. Esthetic Dentistry Research Group, eds: *Reality*. Houston: Reality Publishing Co.; 1993.

25. Davis EL, Joynt RB, Yu X, Wieczkowski G Jr: **Dentin bonding system shelf life and bond strength.** *Am J Dent* 1993, **6**:229–231.

26. Kanca J: **Improving bond strength through acid etching of dentin and bonding to wet dentin surfaces.** *J Am Dent Assoc* 1992, **123**:35–43.

27. Lacy AM, Wada C, Du W, Watanabe L: **In vitro microleakage at the gingival margin of porcelain and resin veneers.** *J Prosthet Dent* 1992, **67**:7–10.

28. Tam LE, McComb D: **Shear bond strengths of resin luting cements to laboratory-made composite resin veneers.** *J Prosthet Dent* 1991, **66**:314–321.

29. Stokes AN, Hood JAA: **Impact fracture characteristics of intact and crowned human central incisors.** *J Oral Rehabil* 1993, **20**:89–95.

When teeth were struck on their middle labial surfaces by a pendulum impact device, porcelain veneers were remarkably resistant to impact fracture. Where they did fracture, they fractured at the site of impact but remained cemented. Porcelain veneer fracture patterns were similar to those for intact, unrestored teeth. Dicor crowns were less fracture-resistant than other restoration types tested. Porcelain veneers and full gold crowns stiffened teeth, which led to more root fractures than the porcelain crowns.

30. Monsenego G, Burdairon G, Clerjaud B: **Fluorescence of dental porcelain.** *J Prosthet Dent* 1993, **69**:106–113.

31. Berrong JM, Weed RM, Schwartz IS: **Color stability of selected dual-cure composite resin cements.** *J Prosthodont* 1993, **2**:24–27.

Color changes occurring in thin layers of resin may have less visual effect than similar discoloration occurring in a resin mass of greater thickness. This discoloration would not be as important in multiple veneer cases.

32. Chpindel P, Cristou M: **Tooth preparation and fabrication of porcelain veneers using a double-layer technique.** *Pract Periodontics Aesthet Dent* 1994, **6**:19–30.

The discrepancy between the surface reflection and the internal reflection provides the illusion of transparency. If the internal reflection is greater than the surface reflection, you will have an opaque material; if the internal reflection is less than the surface reflection, you will have a transparent material. The double-layer technique allows the discrepancy between the surface porcelain's increased translucent reflection and the internal porcelain's diminished translucent reflection to give an illusion of transparency that compares favorably with that of natural teeth.

33. Triolo PT Jr, Swift EJ Jr, Judgil A, Levine A: **Effects of etching time on enamel bond strengths.** *Am J Dent* 1993, **6**:302–304.

Recommends etching the enamel, dentin, and cementum with 30% to 40% phosphoric acid for 15 to 20 seconds.

34. Perdigao J, Denehy GE, Swift EJ Jr: **Effects of chlorhexidine on dentin surfaces and shear bond strengths.** *Am J Dent* 1994, **7**:81–84.

35. Dietschi D, Magne P, Holz J: **An in vitro study of parameters related to marginal and internal seal of bonded restorations.** *Quintessence Int* 1993, 24:281–291.

No statistically significant differences were found among the diverse cement thicknesses (indicating that you can remove extra discolored dentin from heavily stained areas, which will allow thicker cement to mask highly discolored areas) or the luting agents evaluated. When polymerization forces exceed the adhesion of the cement to the substrate and the plastic or elastic deformation of the system, adhesive or cohesive fractures will occur. Actually, the main limitations of adhesive restorations to date have been the insufficient dentinal bonding in clinical conditions related to thin gingival enamel margins. Adhesive fractures on dentin or near the cementoenamel junction will lead to marginal or internal leakage, which is responsible for dentinal pain, recurrent caries, and injuries to the pulp.

36. Freedman G: **Imperva: a bond for all reasons.** *Am Acad Cosmetic Dent J* 1994, Special commemorative issue (adhesion synopsis): 13–14.

37. Feigenbaum NL: **Dentin bonding agents: is there a difference?** *Am Acad Cosmetic Dent J* 1994, Special commemorative issue (adhesion synopsis): 10–11.

38. Miyajima K, Shirakawa K, Senda A: **Application of porcelain veneers following orthodontic treatment.** *J Can Dent Assoc* 1993, 59:167–170.

Bonded porcelain veneer restorations show an 8-year clinical recall success rate between 95% and 97% at the University of Western Ontario and the University of Manitoba. As bonding materials and veneer restoration techniques have improved, functional demand has now been accepted and can be applied to compensate for the limitations of orthodontic treatment.

39. Bona AD, Barghi N: **Removal of partially or fully polymerized resin from porcelain veneers.** *J Prosthet Dent* 1993, 69:443–444.

After a try-in of multiple units, the overhead lights, the dental unit light, or both may initiate polymerization of the resin. Nonpolymerized resin is easily removed with a solvent such as acetone or partially or fully polymerized resin. A debonded veneer does not dissolve in acetone and must be removed by other methods.

40. Knight GT, Berry TG, Barghi N, Burns TR: **Effects of two methods of moisture control on marginal microleakage between resin composite and etched enamel: a clinical study.** *Int J Prosthodont* 1993, 6:475–479.

41. Leinfelder K: **Current developments in dentin bonding systems.** *J Am Dent Assoc* 1993, 123:40–42.

42. Cavanaugh RR, Croll TP: **Bonded porcelain veneer masking of dark tetracycline dentinal stains.** *Pract Periodontics Aesthet Dent* 1994, 6:71–79.

43. Chan KC, Swift EJ Jr: **Marginal seal of new-generation dental bonding agents.** *J Prosthet Dent* 1994, 72:420–423.

44. Thurmond JW, Barkmeier WW, Wilwerding TM: **Effect of porcelain surface treatments on bond strengths of composite resin bonded to porcelain.** *J Prosthet Dent* 1994, 72:355–359.

45. Denissen HW, Wijnhoff GFA, Veldhuis AAH, Kalk W: **Five-year study of all-porcelain veneer fixed partial dentures.** *J Prosthet Dent* 1993, 69:464–468.

A 75% success rate with 12 porcelain veneer fixed partial dentures after 5 years is reported.

Frederick W. Costello, DDS, 1089 West Granada Boulevard, #1 Ormond Beach, FL 32174, USA.

Advances in adhesive technology

T. Gary Alex, DMD

Huntington, New York, USA

Advances in adhesive technology have occurred at a remarkable pace over the past few years. It seems as though every month brings a "new" and "better" bonding system onto the market. Clinical protocol is constantly changing. Just when clinicians have mastered one technique, they find it has been supplanted by another. This often creates confusion and suspicion on the part of the dental practitioner. There are, however, some fundamental concepts applicable to almost all adhesive systems. This paper attempts to present a lucid and comprehensible review of some of these concepts. Many of the latest innovations, such as total etch and wet bonding, are discussed. This paper is not intended as a comprehensive review of all aspects of adhesive dentistry. (For example, adhesion to metals is not covered.) It is my hope that readers will come away with a basic understanding of some current concepts and beliefs in the constantly evolving field of adhesive dentistry.

In the fourteenth century, Europe emerged from the Dark Ages via the Renaissance. This emergence encompassed not only art, science, and literature, but more profoundly, thought itself. The genesis of new ideas and concepts forever changed humanity's view of the universe. What had been considered impossible was now possible. That which had been unthinkable was now a lucid thought with limitless possibilities. In a very real sense, we are in the midst of a Renaissance in adhesive dentistry. The concepts of total etch [1,2], wet dentin bonding [3], and hybrid layer formation [4,5] were unthinkable and incomprehensible just a short time ago. Through the dedication and insight of individuals like those who first described these concepts, we are, in a sense, emerging from the dark ages of adhesion and into a new era.

When I was approached to write this review article on adhesion for *Current Opinion in Cosmetic Dentistry*, I was asked to focus on advances and improvements in adhesive technology over the past 2 years. This request is somewhat analogous to reading only the last chapter of a great novel. You understand where you are now, but have no idea how you arrived there. To comprehend the present, it is necessary to review the past briefly.

Enamel bonding

In 1955, Buonocore [6] introduced a revolutionary technique for bonding acrylic resins to enamel surfaces. He found that if he treated the enamel surface with phosphoric acid, the restorative resins subsequently placed adhered more durably to the tooth structure. The elucidation of this interaction by Gwinnett and Buonocore [7] was the first step in the modern adhesive story. Subsequent research, clinical observation, and anecdotal evidence established the reliability of the bond to acid-etched enamel.

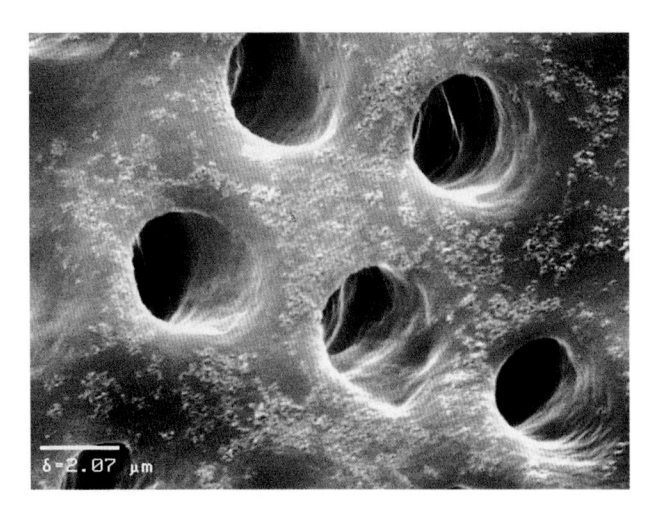

Fig. 1. Scanning electron microscope image of silica residue on the dentin surface after conditioning with traditional 37% phosphoric acid gel. (*Courtesy of* A. J. Gwinnett, Stony Brook, NY.)

Several significant changes have recently taken place regarding the acid etching (*ie*, conditioning) of enamel surfaces. These include the development of gel and "semigel" etching agents, a reduction in the acid application time, and the use of acid conditioners other than traditional phosphoric acid (*ie*, nitric, citric, oxalic, maleic acids). Phosphoric acid gels were developed to give the clinician a greater degree of control and precision in the placement of etching agents. Most conventional gel etchants use submicron silica as a thickening agent, which affords the needed viscosity that characterizes them as a "gel." Etching gels are frequently used in this country for the simultaneous etching of the enamel and conditioning of dentin surfaces (the "total etch" technique). Some researchers have observed that even after these gels are rinsed off, a silica residue (Fig. 1) can be seen in microscopic examination of the dentin [8–10]. The question is, does this residue, which can be considered a surface contaminant, in any way interfere with the adhesive abilities of current bonding systems? The literature is equivocal on this question. Some studies suggested that this silica residue may adversely affect the bonding abilities of some dentin bonding systems [11•,12]. Other studies found little difference in bond strengths whether the etching gel used contains silica or not [13]. Gwinnett (Personal communication) found no difference in bond strengths to ground and unground enamel surfaces using acids with and without a silica matrix. Suh [14], chemist and founder of the Bisco Corporation (Itasca, IL), was, to my best knowledge, the first to develop non–silica containing semigels. These semigels, now used by several manufacturers, employ polymeric thickening agents. They apparently leave no debris on the surface, may have better wetting abilities, and rinse off more easily than conventional silica-containing gels. Suh went one step further by incorporating the antibacterial agent benzalkonium chloride in his semigel formulation. Chan [15,16] showed that even after rinsing, the benzalkonium chloride incorporated into this semigel etchant exhibited significant antimicrobial properties. Residual benzalkonium chloride has been shown to have no adverse effects on the bonding abilities of the All-Bond 2 (Bisco) dentin bonding system [17•]. According to the hypothesis of Brannstrom et al. [18,19], bacterial irritation is the main cause of pulpal damage beneath silicate, acrylic, and composite restorations. Therefore, the development of antibacterial conditioning formulations may be a significant step in improving the long-term clinical expectations of bonded restorations.

Another recent trend relating to acid conditioning of enamel surfaces is reduction of etching time and acid concentration. The standard treatment protocol for the etching of enamel surfaces has been 37% phosphoric acid applied for 60 seconds. Several studies show no difference in shear bond strength of materials bonded to enamel etched with 37% phosphoric acid for 15 or 60 seconds [20–22]. The microscopic appearance of the enamel also shows essentially no difference in etch pattern at either application time [21,23••]. Manufacturers are decreasing the concentration of phosphoric acid as well as decreasing etching time. A comparison of different etching times and different phosphoric acid concentrations shows no statistically significant differences in the shear bond strength in permanent and primary teeth [24,25]. Commercially available products currently include concentrations of phosphoric acid that range from 10% to 50%. The etching of enamel at lower concentrations and shorter application times may be significant when total etch bonding techniques are employed.

The term *total etch*, first described by Fusayama et al. [1], refers to simultaneous acidic treatment of enamel and dentin surfaces, which offers a clinical advantage, because a single step simultaneously conditions both tissues [23••]. Excessive demineralization of the dentin should be avoided in this technique, because bond strength may be compromised. Lower concentrations of phosphoric acid and reduced etching times that give an adequate etch of the enamel while avoiding excessive demineralization of the dentin are desirable. I recommend etching times of 15 seconds for 32% or 37% phosphoric acid, and 25 to 30 seconds for 10% phosphoric acid.

Recently, acids other then phosphoric have been employed in commercially available adhesive systems. These include nitric, maleic, oxalic, and citric acid. When they are used in a total etch capacity, however, there has been some question as to their ability to etch enamel as capably as phosphoric acid [26,27•,28]. Other studies demonstrated little difference between these acids and traditional phosphoric acid in terms of enamel etching ability [29–31]. Because the literature is equivocal, it may be wise to use traditional phosphoric acid for total etch procedures. A word of caution is in order, however. Some adhesive systems, such as Amalgambond (Parkell, Farmingdale, NY), do not perform as well when phosphoric acid is substituted for the citric acid and ferric chloride formulation that comes with the kit [32•]. Unless you know exactly what you are doing, it is prudent to follow the manufacturer's instructions.

Dentin bonding

Although enamel has proven a reliable substrate for bonding, bonding to dentin is less reliable and predictable. This is due largely to the morphologic, histologic, and compositional differences between the two substrates. The inorganic content of mature enamel amounts to 96% to 97% hydroxyapatite (by weight). The remainder is water and organic material [33•]. These percentages remain generally consistent throughout the enamel. On the other hand, dentin is approximately 70% hydroxyapatite (by weight), 18% organic material (mainly collagen), and 12% water [33•]. These percentages are not consistent and can vary significantly depending on a number of factors including dentin depth, the age of the teeth, and history of tooth trauma or pathology. Superficial, middle, and deep dentin surfaces can be quite different in their structural and chemical composition. These differences, coupled with the relatively high water content of dentin, present a challenge to consistent and

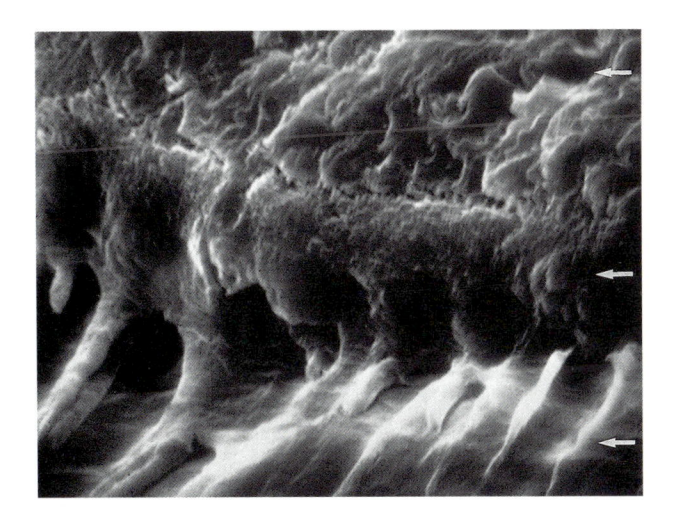

Fig. 2. Scanning electron microscope image of hybrid (resin-reinforced) layer. *Top arrow* indicates resin. *Middle arrow* indicates hybrid zone. *Bottom arrow* indicates dentin. (*Courtesy of* A. J. Gwinnett, Stony Brook, NY.)

reliable bonding. The ideal dentin-enamel bonding system as described by Kanca [34••] should provide gap-free composite restorations, achieve rapidly developing high bond strengths, be biocompatible, function in the presence of moisture, and treat dentin and enamel simultaneously.

Producing gap-free restorations is especially important because it helps minimize microleakage. All of the current polymeric composite restorative resins shrink during polymerization, resulting in the development of tensile stress, shear stress, or both at the tooth-restoration interface [35•]. This, coupled with differences in coefficients of thermal expansion between tooth structure and the restorative material, water sorption, and occlusal load, can lead to gaps and microleakage. Some studies, done with the latest generation of adhesive systems, showed that microleakage was significantly reduced but not eliminated at the dentin-restoration interface [35•,36,37]. Gwinnett and Kanca [38••] were the first to demonstrate gap-free composite restorations *in vivo* using a total etch technique in conjunction with an acetone-containing primer system. Their results were confirmed by Gwinnett *et al.* [39••].

Total etch

Total etch procedures have gained in popularity over the last few years, and for good reason. As mentioned, dentin and enamel can be treated in one step, which saves time and reduces the potential for operator error. It is my observation that almost all adhesive systems are becoming total etch systems, some using phosphoric acid, some using other acids. Acid removes the dentin smear layer, raises surface energy, and modifies the dentin substrate so that it can be infiltrated by subsequently placed primers and resins. Up until re-

cently, the intentional placement of acids on dentin, especially phosphoric acid, was considered taboo. It was believed that applying phosphoric acid to the dentin would harm the pulp. Concerns about acid etching of dentin derived largely from studies conducted 20 years ago by Macko *et al.* [40], Retief *et al.* [41], and Stanley *et al.* [42]. It was concluded from these studies that phosphoric acid treatment of dentin had a deleterious effect on the pulp. These conclusions were challenged in 1985 by Bertolotti [43], who was the first to advocate the use of total etch in this country. His work was based on concepts developed by Fusayama *et al.* [1] in Japan in the late 1970s. Kanca [44•] then offered an alternative hypothesis to the conclusions of the earlier studies. He hypothesized that the previously reported pulpal responses were caused by prolonged exposure to zinc oxide and particularly to eugenol (a phenol), and not to phosphoric acid. Recent studies by Cox *et al.* [45••,46•] strongly support Kanca's hypothesis. In any case, total etch procedures are employed by a significant number of clinicians with excellent success.

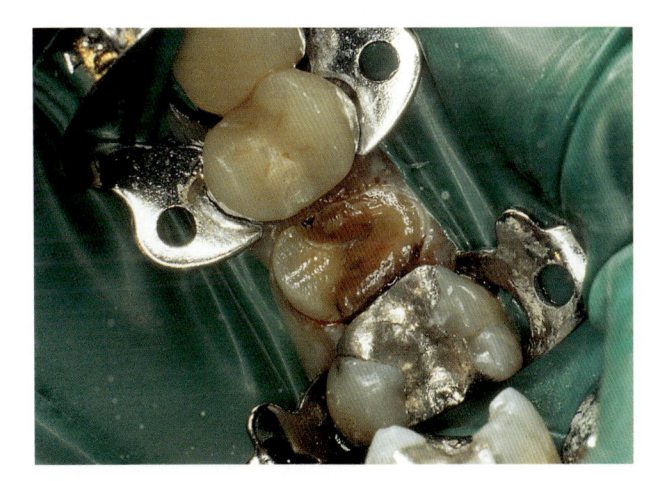

Fig. 3. Clinical appearance of a dentin surface well primed with the All-Bond 2 bonding system (Bisco, Itasca, IL). The primer has been completely air-dried. The hybrid layer is formed at this stage.

Hybrid layer

One of the reasons for this success is the ability of hydrophilic resin primers in current adhesive systems to penetrate acid demineralized dentin and form a "hybrid" layer. The hybrid layer, first described by Nakabayashi *et al.* [47], is a thin layer (approximately 2 to 6 µm) of resin-infiltrated dentin (Figs. 2 and 3). This layer provides an important seal that protects the dentin and pulp. The thickness and quality of the hybrid layer vary depending on the bonding system and the technique employed. Many primers in current adhesive systems are incorporated into acetone or alcohol, which acts as a solvent. This is significant because both acetone and alcohol have excellent "wetting" properties as well as a natural affinity for wa-

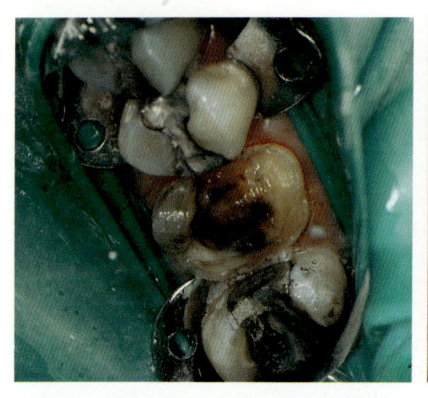

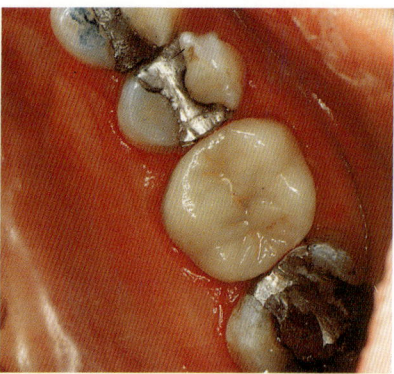

Fig. 4. Left, A tooth prior to restoration with a laboratory-processed composite onlay. At one time, a tooth such as this could be restored only with full coverage and possible endodontic intervention. **Right**, Completed onlay restoration bonded in with a total etch, wet bonding technique.

ter. This affinity is partially mediated by the ability of these solvents to hydrogen-bond to water molecules. These solvent-primer solutions infiltrate the acid-conditioned dentin, where the solvents subsequently evaporate, leaving the primer behind. The primers then polymerize by a self- or light-cure mechanism, or both. Curing micromechanically locks them into the dentin substrate, forming the hybrid layer. Subsequently placed bonding resins and composites chemically bond to this layer via pendant methacrylate groups. Some believe that the hybrid layer and not resin penetration into the dentin tubules is the main factor responsible for the bond strengths of the latest adhesive systems [48]. The reader is referred to recent studies by Gwinnett *et al.* [39••] and Van Meerbeek *et al.* [49••,50••] for excellent descriptions of the physical and chemical nature of hybrid layer formation.

Wet bonding

Another important recent innovation is the concept of wet bonding. Kanca [3] found that the presence of moisture on the dentin substrate, prior to primer application, significantly enhanced the bonding capabilities of some adhesive systems. This process has come to be called *wet dentin bonding* (although *moist dentin bonding* may be a more accurate description). Kanca's findings were confirmed in two recent studies [32•,51•]. Once again, it is the extreme hydrophilic (water-loving) nature of the primer-solvent mixture that helps explain its ability to function optimally in a moist environment. Caution is in order, however, because some systems are not amenable to this technique. (Once again, follow the manufacturer's instructions.)

Ideally, the aim of a dentin bonding protocol should be to condition the tissue, disinfect it, and produce a seal through a bond between the tissue and resin based restoratives. There are many commercial products, such as Tubulicid (Global Dental, North Bellmore, NY), Concepsis (Ultradent Products, Salt Lake City, UT), and Cavity Cleanser (Bisco), that can be used to disinfect preparations prior to or in conjunction with adhesive restorative procedures. Some current adhesive systems achieve bond strengths to dentin that equal or surpass bond strengths to etched enamel (20 MPa or better). Bond strength values such as these are believed adequate enough to overcome polymerization shrinkage associated with resin restoratives [52]. As mentioned, gap-free composite restorations have been demonstrated *in vivo*. Ample evidence suggests that because of their biocompatibility and sealing capability, new adhesive systems should take the place of conventional bases and liners such as calcium hydroxide [53••]. In fact, traditional bases and liners are contraindicated because they physically interfere with what dentin bonding agents are designed to do, *ie*, interact with the dentin and the surface area that this tissue offers in the bonding process.

Conclusions

Cavity disinfection, total etch, wet bonding, and hybrid layer formation have been shown to effectively seal the dentin, minimize microleakage, and virtually eliminate postoperative sensitivity. Such achievements strongly encourage the dentist of today to reevaluate his or her restorative techniques, especially regarding the conservation of tooth structure. Laboratory-processed composite or porcelain onlays can now be bonded confidently on teeth once restorable only with full coverage [54•] (Fig. 4). The effectiveness of porcelain laminates bonded to anterior teeth with appropriate adhesive systems is well documented [55,56]. Extensive tooth preparation to allow for resistance and retention form has been minimized or eliminated. The need to routinely place posts after endodontic treatment is no longer necessary. Adhesive restorations conserve, support, and strengthen tooth tissue and thus help to preserve the biologic and biophysical properties of the tooth.

Although, the renaissance in adhesive dentistry is indeed upon us, much research has yet to be done. Improvements and refinements will continue in the future. Used in a knowledgeable fashion, with attention to technique and materials, current adhesive technology can offer expanded treatment options and lead the clinician confidently into restorative techniques previously considered impossible. The implications for the dental profession, patients, and the individual practitioner are fantastic.

References and recommended reading

Papers of particular interest, published within the annual period of review, have been highlighted as:
- • Of special interest
- •• Of outstanding interest

1. Fusayama T, Nakamura M, Kurosaki N, Iwaku M: **Nonpressure adhesion of a new adhesive restorative resin.** *J Dent Res* 1979, **58**:1364–1370.

2. Fusayama T: **Total etch technique and cavity isolation.** *J Esthet Dent* 1992, **4**:105–109.

3. Kanca J III: **Effect of drying on bond strength [abstract].** *J Dent Res* 1991, **70**:20.

4. Nakabayashi N: **Resin reinforced dentin due to infiltration of monomers into the dentin at the adhesive interface.** *J Jpn Dent Mater* 1982, **16**:78–81.

5. Gwinnett AJ, Matsui A: **A study of enamel adhesives: the physical relationship between enamel and adhesive.** *Arch Oral Biol* 1967, **23**:1615–1619.

6. Buonocore MG: **A simple method of increasing the adhesion of acrylic filling materials to enamel surfaces.** *J Dent Res* 1955, **34**:849–853.

7. Gwinnett AJ, Buonocore MG: **Adhesives and caries prevention: a preliminary study.** *Br Dent J* 1965, **119**:77–80.

8. Kubo S, Finger W, Mueller M, Podszun W: **Principals and mechanism of bonding with dentin adhesive materials.** *J Esthet Dent* 1991, **3**:62–69.

9. Suh BI: **All-Bond: fourth generation dentin bonding system.** *J Esthet Dent* 1991, **3**:139–147.

10. Fujitani M, Inokoshi S, Hosoda H: **Effect of acid etching on the dental pulp in adhesive composite restorations.** *Int Dent J* 1992, **42**:3–11.

11. Kanca J III: **Etchant composition and bond strength to**
• **dentin.** *Am J Dent* 1993, **6**:287–290.
Innovative study comparing silica-containing gels with nonsilica semigel formulations and the effect on bond strength of various adhesive systems.

12. Kanca J III: **The effect of etchants on bond strength to dentin [abstract].** *J Dent Res* 1993, **72**:136.

13. Myers M, Dickinson G, Hoyle S: **Effect of a silica-containing etchant on shear bond strength to dentin.** *Pract Periodontics Aesthet Dent* 1993, **5**:45–48.

14. Suh BI: **All-Bond: fourth generation dentin bonding system.** *J Esthet Dent* 1991, **3**:139–147.

15. Chan DCN, Hui E: **Antimicrobial action of chlorhexidine incorporated in an etchant [abstract].** *J Dent Res* 1992, **71**(special issue):284.

16. Chan DCN, Lo W: **Antimicrobial action of benzalkonium chloride-containing etchant.** *J Dent Res* 1994, **73**(special issue):995.

17. Gwinnett AJ: **Effect of cavity disinfection on bond strength**
• **to dentin.** *J Esthet Dent* 1992, **4**(special issue):11–13.
Concise study demonstrating the effect of two disinfecting agents on the bonding abilities of the All-Bond 2 adhesive system. Well-written and to the point.

18. Brannstrom M, Nyborg H: **Cavity treatment with a microbiocidal fluoride solution: growth of bacteria and effect on the pulp.** *J Prosthet Dent* 1973, **30**:303–310.

19. Brannstrom M, Vojinoric O, Nordenvall K: **Bacterial and pulpal reactions under silicate cement restorations.** *J Prosthet Dent* 1979, **41**:290–295.

20. Sheen DH, Wang WN, Tarng TH: **Bond strength of younger and older permanent teeth with various etching times.** *Angle Orthod* 1993, **63**:225–230.

21. Barkmeier WW, Shaffer SE, Gwinnett AJ: **Effects of 15 vs 60 second enamel acid conditioning on adhesion and morphology.** *Oper Dent* 1986, **11**:111–116.

22. Nordenvall KJ, Brannstrom M, Malmgren O: **Etching of deciduous teeth and young and old permanent teeth.** *Am J Orthod* 1980, **78**:99–108.

23. Gwinnett AJ: **Bonding basics: what every clinician should**
•• **know.** *Esthet Dent Update* 1994, **5**:35–41.
A well-written historical and contemporary overview by one of the giants in the field, and a must read for anyone interested in adhesive dentistry. Adhesion to enamel and dentin is described in a concise and comprehensible fashion. Up to date and right on the mark.

24. Garcia-Godoy F, Gwinnett AJ: **Effect of etching times and mechanical pretreatment of the enamel of primary teeth.** *Am J Dent* 1991, **4**:115–119.

25. Sheen DH, Wang WN, Tarng TH: **Bond strength of younger and older permanent teeth with various etching times.** *Angle Orthod* 1993, **63**:225–230.

26. Joynt RB, Davis EL, Yu XY: **Adhesion of direct restorative materials.** *N Y State Dent J* 1992, June/July:41–45.

27. Swift EJ, Denehy GE, Beck MD: **Use of phosphoric acid**
• **etchants with Scotchbond Multi-Purpose.** *Am J Dent* 1993, **6**:88–90.
Swift has written several fine papers on Scotchbond Multi-Purpose adhesive (3M Dental Products, St. Paul, MN). This paper evaluates the dentin bond strengths of Multi-Purpose when a phosphoric acid agent, 10% maleic acid, or Etch and Seal (Den-Mat, Santa Maria, CA) is used as the dentin conditioner.

28. Swift EJ, Cloe BC: **Shear bond strengths of new enamel etchants.** *Am J Dent* 1993, **6**:162–164.

29. Saunders WP, Strang R, Ahmad I: **Shear bond strength of mirage bond to enamel and dentin.** *Am J Dent* 1991, **4**:265–267.

30. Nakabayashi N: **Resin reinforced dentin due to infiltration of monomers into the dentin at the adhesive interface.** *J Jpn Dent Mater* 1982, **16**:78–81.

31. Swift EJ, Triolo PT: **Bond strength of scotchbond multipurpose to moist dentin and enamel.** *Am J Dent* 1992, **5**:318–320.

32. Perdigao J, Swift EJ, Cloe BC: **Effects of etchants, surface**
• **moisture, and resin composite on dentin bond strengths.** *Am J Dent* 1993, **6**:61–64.
In vitro study that evaluates effects of etchant type, surface moisture, and resin composite type on the shear bond strength of dentin adhesives. All-Bond 2, Amalgambond, and Clearfil Photo Bond (Kuraray Co., Tokyo, Japan) are evaluated. A well-written, clear, and concise report.

33. Van Meerbeek B, Lambrechts P, Inokoshi S, Braem M, Vanherle G: **Factors affecting adhesion to mineralized tissues.**
• *Oper Dent* 1992, **5**(suppl):111–124.
This paper is an excellent review of the literature concerning factors affecting adhesion to mineralized tissues. Well-written and comprehensive.

34. Kanca J III: **Improving bond strength through acid etching**
•• **of dentin and bonding to wet dentin surfaces.** *J Am Dent Assoc* 1992, **123**:35–42.
Well-written and readable account of the wet bonding technique. Rationale and clinical protocol are discussed.

35. Retief DH: **Do adhesives prevent microleakage?** *Int Dent J*
• 1994, **44**:19–26.

Retief has been studying adhesive dentistry for a long time. This informative paper describes microleakage studies of various adhesive systems. The cautious Retief has some important things to say.

36. Mandras RS, Retief DH, Russell CM: **Quantitative microleakage of six dentin bonding systems.** *Am J Dent* 1993, 6:119–122.

37. Sidhu SK, Henderson LJ: **Dentin adhesives and microleakage in cervical resin composites.** *Am J Dent* 1992, 5:240–244.

38. Gwinnett AJ, Kanca J III: **Micromorphological relationship between resin and dentin in vitro and in vivo.** *Am J Dent* 1992, 5:73–77.
••

This fine study examines the relationship between resin and dentin *in vitro* and *in vivo* using a total etch technique. Gwinnett and Kanca were the first to demonstrate a gap-free composite restoration *in vivo*.

39. Gwinnett AJ, Tay FR, Pang KM, Wei SHY: **Structural evidence of a sealed tissue interface with a total-etch wet-bonding technique in vivo.** *J Dent Res* 1994, 73:629–636.
••

The first *in vivo* study to characterize the hybrid layer in deep, vital, human dentin with light microscopy, scanning electron microscopy, and transmission electron microscopy. This study investigates the resin-dentin interface of *in vivo* specimens restored with the All-Bond 2 adhesive system by use of a total etch, wet bonding technique. Just a fantastic paper with superb microscopic photographs and illustrations.

40. Macko D, Rutberg M, Langeland K: **Pulpal response to the application of phosphoric acid to dentin.** *Oral Surg Oral Med Oral Pathol* 1978, 45:930–946.

41. Retief D, Austin J, Fatti L: **Pulpal response to phosphoric acid.** *J Oral Pathol Med* 1974, 3:114–22.

42. Stanley H, Going R, Chauncey H: **Human pulp response to acid pretreatment of dentin and to composite restoration.** *J Am Dent Assoc* 1975, 91:817–825.

43. Bertolotti R: **1992: the year of total etch.** *Adhesive Dentistry Newsletter* December 1992:1–6.

44. Kanca J III: **An alternative hypothesis to the cause of pulpal inflammation in teeth treated with phosphoric acid on dentin.** *Quintessence Int* 1990, 21:83–86.
•

Another well-written paper by Kanca exploring the possible causes of pulpal sensitivity.

45. Cox CF: **Effects of adhesive resins and various dental cements on the pulp.** *Oper Dent* 1992, 5(suppl):165–176.
••

Superb study that makes the reader question many current beliefs about what contributes to pulpal damage and sensitivity after restorative procedures.

46. Cox CF, Snuggs HM, Powell CS, White KC: **Pulpal healing and dentinal bridge formation in an acidic environment.** *Quintessence Int* 1993, 24:501–510.
•

This study is designed to observe the healing and bridging capacity of mechanically exposed pulps capped with various acidic cements. Results show the acidic cements resulted in pulpal healing similar to that seen in controls treated with calcium hydroxide.

47. Nakabayashi N, Kojima K, Masuhara E: **The promotion of adhesion by the infiltration of monomers into tooth substrates.** *J Biomed Mater Res* 1982, 16:265–273.

48. Erickson RL: **Surface interactions of dentin adhesive materials.** *Oper Dent* 1992, 5(suppl):81–94.

49. Van Meerbeek B, Dhem A, Goret-Nicaise M, Braem M, Lambrechts P, Vanherle G: **Comparative SEM and TEM examination of the ultrastructure of the resin-dentin interdiffusion zone.** *J Dent Res* 1993, 72:495–501.
••

This paper contains some of the finest scanning and transmission electron microscope photographs of the hybrid layer I have ever seen. The morphology of the hybrid layer is explained in detail. One of the best studies of its kind.

50. Van Meerbeek B, Mohrbacher H, Celis JP, Roos JR, Braem M, Lambrechts P, Vanherle G: **Chemical characterization of the resin-dentin interface by micro-Raman spectroscopy.** *J Dent Res* 1993, 72:1423–1428.
••

This study uses micro-Raman spectroscopy to characterize the chemical nature of the interface between dentin and adhesive resin materials. Somewhat technical but very significant and well-written.

51. Gwinnett AJ: **Moist versus dry dentin: its effect on shear bond strength.** *Am J Dent* 1992, 5:127–129.
•

Excellent and well-written paper that confirms the effectiveness of wet bonding with specific adhesive systems.

52. Davidson CL, DeGee AJ, Feilzer AJ: **The competition between the composite dentin bond strength and the polymerization contraction stress.** *J Dent Res* 1984, 63:1396–1399.

53. Cox CF, Suzuki S: **Re-evaluating pulp protection: calcium hydroxide liners vs. cohesive hybridization.** *J Am Dent Assoc* 1994, 124:823–831.
••

Cox has done fantastic work at the University of Alabama, and here, with the help of Suzuki, he has written one of his best papers. Presented for the general dentist in a comprehensible fashion, it questions conventional opinions regarding the effectiveness of bases and liners.

54. Jackson RD: **Esthetic inlays and onlays.** *Curr Opin Cosmetic Dent* 1994, 2:30–39.
•

This very well written paper summarizes scientific and clinical opinion regarding the placement of esthetic inlays and onlays. Rationale for placement and clinical technique are described in detail.

55. Nathanson D, Strassler HE: **Clinical evaluation of etched porcelain veneers over a period of 18-42 months.** *J Esthet Dent* 1989, 1:21–28.

56. Christensen GJ: **Clinical observations of porcelain veneers: a three year report.** *J Esthet Dent* 1991, 3:173–179.

T. Gary Alex, 90 Cove Road, Huntington, NY 11743, USA.

The high-tech dental office

Mark E. Ellicson, DMD

Dalton, Massachusetts, USA

The 1990s ushered in technologic advances affecting the forefront of dentistry. This technology was the harbinger of a change in dentistry from a *need*-driven to a *want*-driven profession. As the twenty-first century approaches, dentistry is embracing these novel advances. Concurrently, the multifarious high-technology equipment brings with it the responsibility for the dentist to educate patients about potential dental benefits that can further enhance their overall health.

In the early 1980s, words such as *CAD-CAM, laser, radiovisiography, electronic claims, bar code scanning, intra- and extraoral computer imaging, electronic anesthesia, virtual reality glasses, voice recognition,* and *multimedia* were not part of our vocabulary. Now, as we approach the midpoint of this decade, these terms are commonplace. The benefits realized from the utilization of these advances reside in the changing attitudes of our educated patients toward their needs and wants. No longer does it suffice to treat only the functional aspects of dental health; rather, the cosmetic result is very much a consideration. Teeth that look pleasing have great appeal, and because of the expeditious means by which healthy teeth can be transformed without damage, esthetic dentistry becomes a *want* [1•,2••].

The present

The dentist of the twenty-first century will continue to be bombarded by the technologic revolution (Fig. 1). The progressive dentist will face a plethora of technologies from which to choose to perform dentistry more efficiently and with desired esthetic results. The concept of *total system integration* allows the dentist to share and utilize patient information easily throughout the dental office (Fig. 2) [3••]. Furthermore, the inclusion of integrative technologies fosters a holistic approach to dental care, because the entire team understands the treatment plan and can communicate it to others. Educating patients about the many possibilities allows them to make informed choices.

New patient visit

The reception of the new patient serves as a welcoming session. The receptionist addresses the patient by name, and any number of salutations follow. The patient is escorted to a private consultation area where the receptionist registers the individual in the computer. This initial encounter with the new patient is critical because it serves either to catalyze or to inhibit the ensuing consultation visit. The interactive exchange that transpires should permit the patient a safe space to pose questions and have them answered in an unhurried manner. Timing and the ability to be nonintrusive are important attributes of the receptionist, who in this case functions ideally as both a sensitive listener and interviewer. Once the registration information is typed into the computer, the patient is asked to sign with a computer pad and stylus, as well as to commit an electronic signature for insurance purposes. With the permission of the patient, a credit check can be obtained to expedite the payment process. A bar code label can be computer-generated and will follow the patient throughout all future visits.

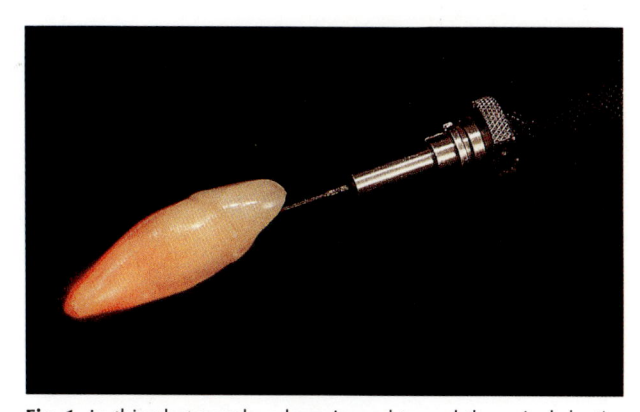

Fig. 1. In this photograph, a laser is used to seal the apical dentin. Laser endodontics is on the verge of reality. (*Courtesy of* American Dental Laser, Troy, MI.)

A dental assistant will then greet and escort the new patient to an operatory. Again, the health history is obtained in an interactive manner. The potential invasiveness of this procedure should be kept in mind. A proficient history taker knows when to sit back and listen, how to pose open-ended, nonthreatening questions, and when to enter the data into the chairside terminal with a light pen on the touch screen.

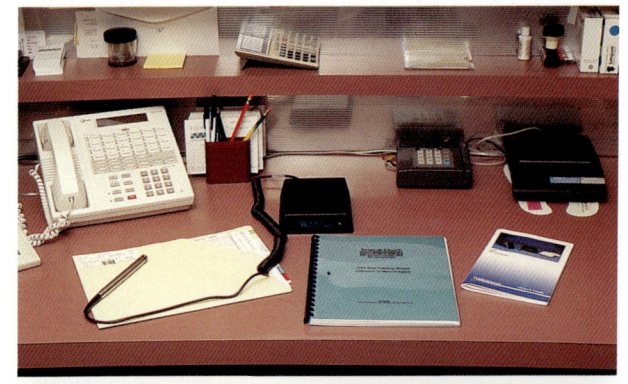

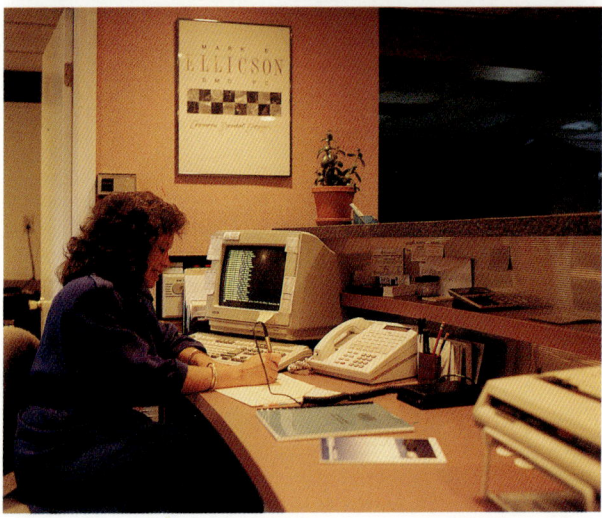

Fig. 2. The tools of the high-tech receptionist include a multiline speaker telephone with voice mail and a digital answering machine, a bar code scanning apparatus, a credit card electronic modem, a computer terminal, and a solar calculator.

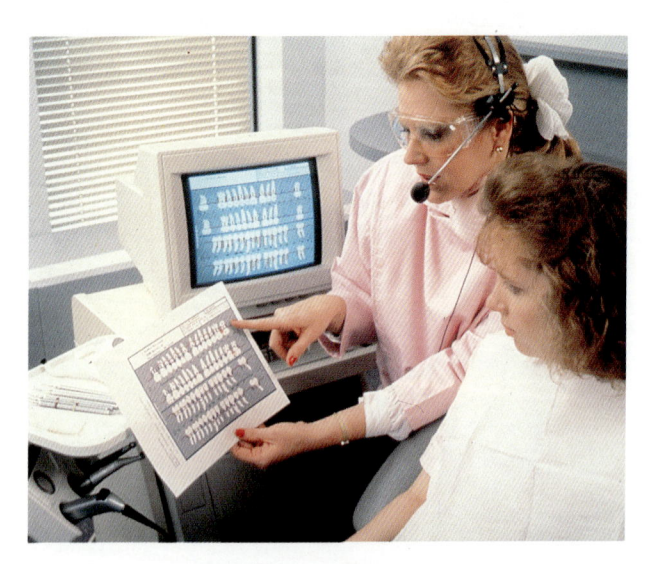

Fig. 3. Patient education with the chairside monitor. (*Courtesy of* Professional Dental Technologies, Batesville, AR.)

The dentist, now the third person to welcome the new patient, spends an unspecified amount of time exploring the patient's understanding of his or her dental needs as well as educating the patient about the realm of dental wants. Patient education tapes, which can provide further visual information about specific treatments, can be seen chairside with or without the dentist (Fig. 3). Many of the procedures are unfamiliar to the patient, and the visual cues given help to clarify them and to generate additional questions.

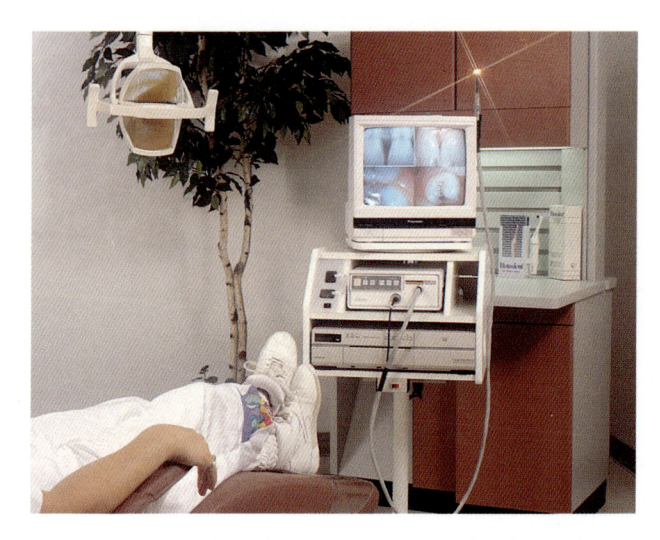

Fig. 4 An intraoral chairside camera. (*Courtesy of* Professional Dental Technologies, Batesville, AR.)

Next, the dentist performs a complete intraoral video examination and generates an extraoral image with a chairside camera (Fig. 4). Periodontal and dental charting are performed with the headset and voice-activated charting function [4], which is aseptic (Fig. 5). After an explanation of its benefits, digital radiovisiography follows. These benefits include reduced cost, less exposure to radiation, an improved image, and instant viewing, and they may improve the patient's understanding and compliance [5••]. Finally, the computer is checked to ascertain whether all information has been entered, the next appointment is scheduled from the interactive scheduling module on the chairside terminal, and the fee for this first visit entered (Fig. 6). This newly entered information is instantly accessible at the receptionist's terminal. The dentist acknowledges the individual's time, patience, and candor and accompanies the patient to the receptionist, who broaches the topic of the fee for that day's treatment. Ideally, the patient is never left unattended throughout the visit.

Diagnosis and treatment plan

Because the terminals are networked, all of the information gleaned during the new-patient visit is available for diagnosis and treatment planning from any terminal in the office (Fig. 7). The treatment plan function allows one to generate insurance forms that can be sent electronically to the various companies, write clinical notes, incorporate periodontal and dental charting, and include intra- and extraoral images. Insurance

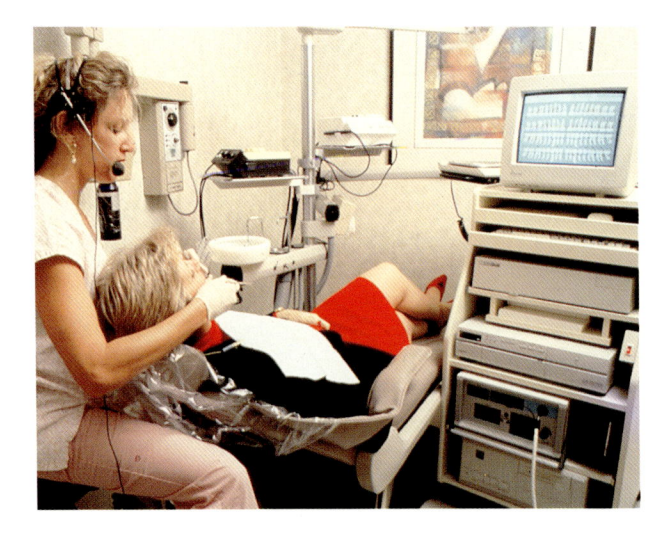

Fig. 5. Voice charting conducted by the hygienist is both hands-free and aseptic. (*Courtesy of* Professional Dental Technologies, Batesville, AR.)

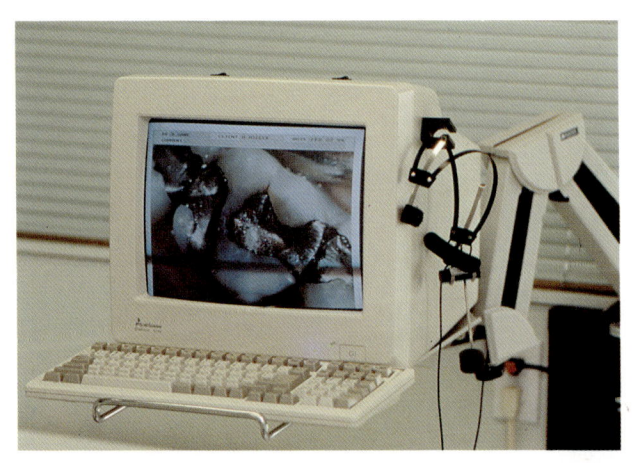

Fig. 6. A chairside monitor on a flexible arm. (*Courtesy of* David Gane, White Rock, BC, Canada.)

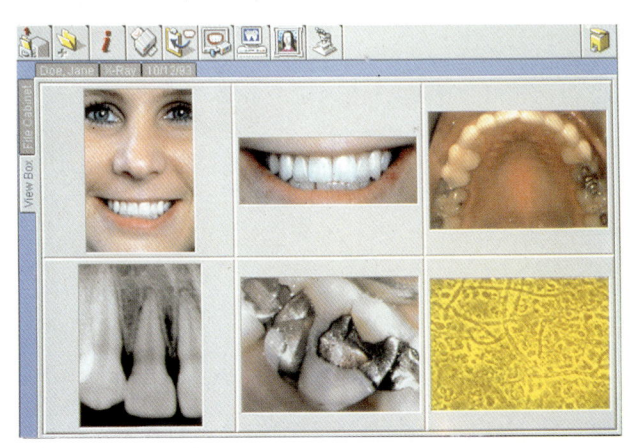

Fig. 7. The information displayed on the chairside monitor includes a full facial image, the smile, an intraoral, occlusal freeze-frame, radiovisiography, intraoral close-up, and phase-contrast microscope slide. (*Courtesy of* D. Gane, White Rock, BC, Canada.)

companies still require radiographs to be printed. The patient's entire record can be printed out for perusal or simply reviewed on the screen at the consultation visit [6••].

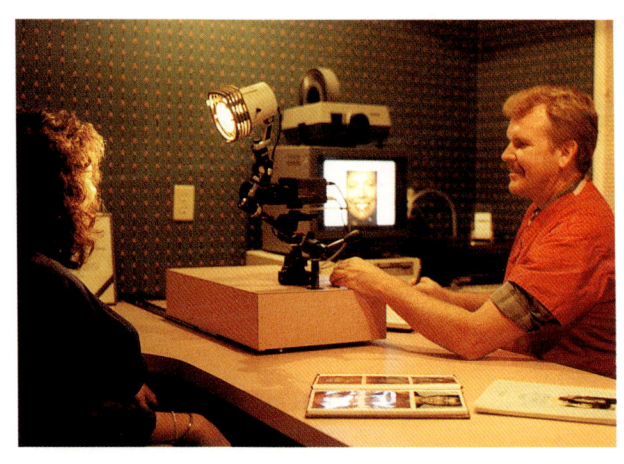

Fig. 8. The imaging and consultation room, which serves as the arena for patient education and conferences.

Consultation visit

At the second office visit, or consultation, the patient is again greeted by the receptionist. Anticipating the patient's arrival, the receptionist has already generated the patient's name and video image. When the patient goes to the private consultation area, the window on the terminal screen depicts the image of the patient made during the initial visit. The chairside terminal also has a window that can signal the patient's arrival by being activated simultaneously. The bar code imprint appears on the care form. The dentist enters and once again greets the patient and the receptionist, allowing the receptionist to exit. All pertinent information is reviewed on the screen, the treatment plan presented, and questions are explored (Fig. 8). The patient is better able to understand an improved image of his or her mouth after having reviewed the intra- and extraoral images that have been digitally enhanced. The amount of time devoted to this consultation visit is individually determined. The dentist gauges time from the cues given by the patient. This exchange should occur in an unrushed and uninterrupted manner. The receptionist returns to review the financial considerations of the treatment plan and then schedules the next appointment. The care form with the bar code is used both to enter the patient information and to serve as a cross reference for balancing out at the end of the day.

Treatment visit

The technology of the 1990s materializes during the first treatment visit. The patient is welcomed and seated in the operatory. Next, the bar code is scanned in,

78   Cosmetic dentistry

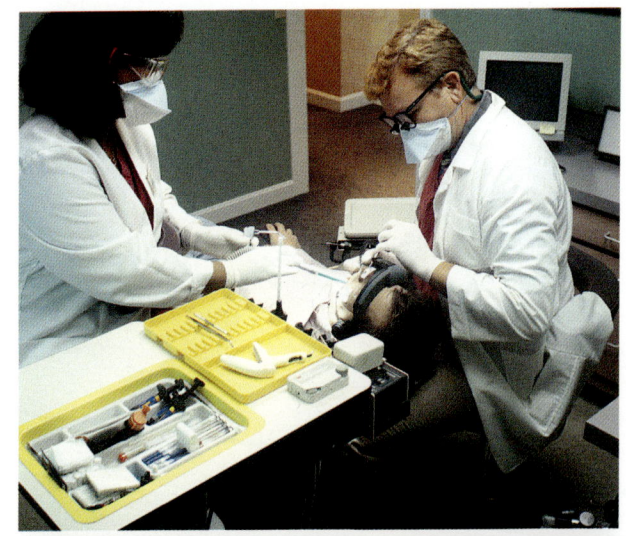

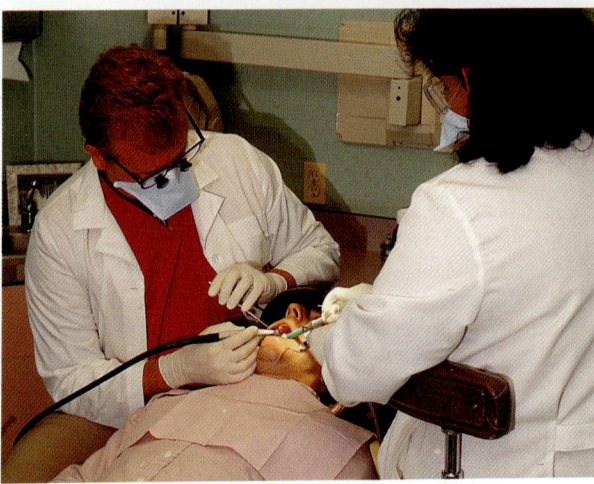

Fig. 9. Top, Virtual reality glasses on a patient. Bottom, Electronic anesthesia is applied to a patient's mandible.

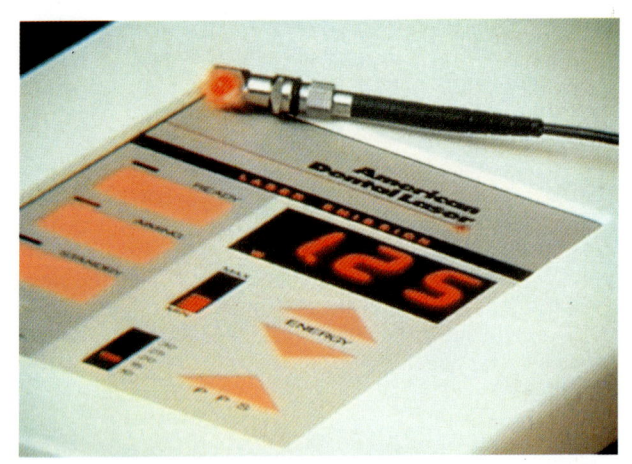

Fig. 10. The laser has revolutionized intraoral soft tissue treatment. (*Courtesy of* American Dental Laser, Troy, MI.)

vision glasses may be donned by the patient and the electronic anesthesia pads applied by the assistant on the mental foramen area of the mandible (Fig. 9) [7]. Topical anesthesia (no needles are used) is administered if needed, and twenty-first century dentistry proceeds. The teeth are prepared, and hemostasis is controlled with a laser (Figs. 10 and 11). The preparation is scanned into a computer, and several inlays are ready to be inserted within a short time (Fig. 12) [8–11]. After the procedure, the patient is asked to comment about the efficacy of the procedure in light of the in-office education received prior to it. The next appointment is made at chairside by the assistant, who then accompanies the patient to the receptionist. The receptionist has the treatment for that visit already on the screen

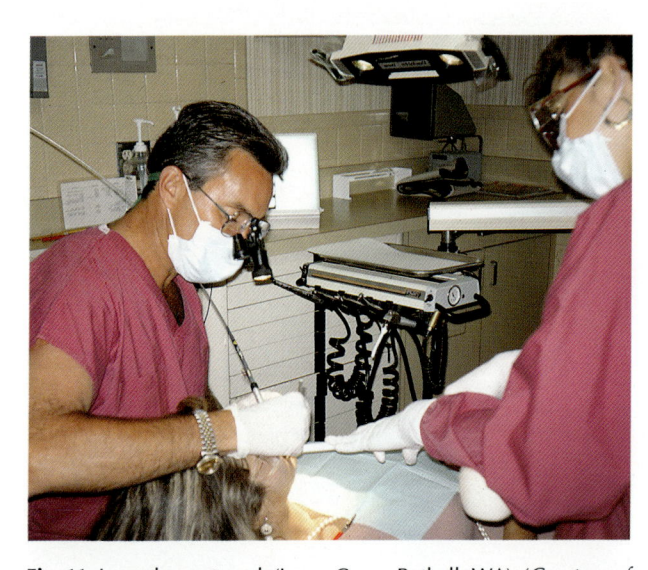

Fig. 11. Luxar laser at work (Luxar Corp., Bothell, WA). (*Courtesy of* G. Ferguson, Upper Montclair, NJ.)

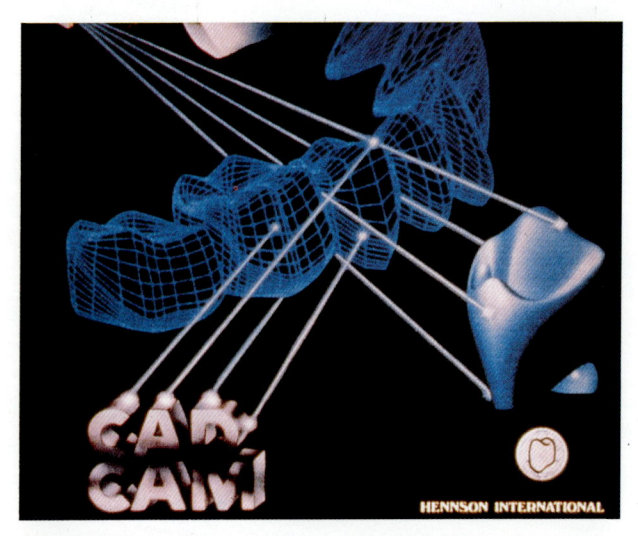

Fig. 12. A computer-generated, three-dimensional wire-form rendering of teeth. Computer-aided design and manufacture (CAD-CAM) provides strong, high-quality restorations in the dentist's office; previously, these achievements were limited to the dental laboratory.

and the patient's dental and periodontal chart, radiograph, and intra- and extraoral images appear. Virtual

and completes the financial aspect of the day's treatment. An electronic insurance form is then generated and sent.

Conclusions

Technology is only a tool. Obviously, the skills necessary to use the tools properly are essential. This technology is changing the nature of dentistry, and as clinicians we are challenged to change with it. Our responsibility remains one of educating patients about these advances to improve the quality of their lives. More important than ever is the need for expert interpersonal skills to maximize this technology.

Acknowledgments

I would like to thank Barbara P. Ellicson of Richmond, Massachusetts and Professional Dental Technologies of Batesville, Arkansas.

References and recommended reading

Papers of particular interest, published within the annual period of review, have been highlighted as:
- Of special interest
- •• Of outstanding interest

1. • Bonner P: **Equipping the complete dental practice.** *Dent Today* 1994, 13:34–41.
This article mentions the high-tech equipment available, including the multimedia armamentarium. The author notes that two doctors always have patient education in mind as they pursue "quality of life dentistry." They cite as their number one priority the communication of knowledge to patients to edify them about what can be offered, and they leave the purchase of unique technology for a well-defined practice up to the dentist.

2. •• Nash R, Nash L, Engelhart D: **New decade dentistry practice development through new technologies.** *Dent Today* 1993, 12:38–42.
This article stresses that proficiency with new technologies is achieved only through continuing education, study, and practice. The entire dental team understands the treatment plan because of video imaging, the use of an intraoral camera, digital radiography, and compact disks. The request for dental services is enhanced by patient education that occurs throughout an office in which dental communication is complete.

3. •• Farr C: **The high-tech practice: a glimpse into the 21st century.** *Dent Today* 1993, 12:32–36.
This writer addresses the shifting paradigms in dentistry and the ethical basis for using high technology, viewing computer networking as a link to sources of clinical information. He also addresses the resistance of some dentists to using the process of electronic insurance claims.

4. Hawley GM, Hamilton FA, Worthington HV: **An investigation into the use of a voice operated data input system.** *Community Dent Oral Epidemiol* 1993, 21:24–26.

5. •• Dunn S, Kantor M: **Digital radiology facts and fictions.** *J Am Dent Assoc* 1993, 124:39–47.
The authors demystify digital radiography, thus enhancing dentists' ability to market the concept to their patients.

6. •• Green S: **Computers are in dentistry's future.** *Dent Econ* 1994, 84:85–88.
A look into the possible technologic future of dentists and their patients.

7. Schazer R, Black R: **Efficacy of electronic dental anesthesia during routine dental operative procedures.** *Gen Dent* 1994, 42:172–176.

8. Pick R, Powell G: **Lasers in dentistry soft-tissue procedures.** *Dent Clin North Am* 1993, 37:281–294.

9. Miller M, Truhe T: **Lasers in dentistry: an overview.** *J Am Dent Assoc* 1993, 124:32–35.

10. White J, Goodis H, Setcos J, Eakle S, Hulscher B, Rose C: **Effects of pulsed Nd:YAG laser energy on human teeth: a three-year follow-up study.** *J Am Dent Assoc* 1993, 124:45–51.

11. Rekow DE: **High technology innovations and limitations for restorative dentistry.** *Dent Clin North Am* 1993, 37: 513–520.

Mark Ellicson, DMD, 227 Main Street, Dalton, MA 01226, USA.

A new esthetic impression system

Laurence R. Rifkin, DDS

Beverly Hills, California, USA

Communication between the restorative dentist and the laboratory technician is essential to establish a predictable esthetic result. Errors in the laboratory can create the need for excessive clinical try-ins and modifications that waste valuable time. This paper reviews the use and potential benefits of a new facial impression system to minimize such esthetic errors. This system provides the laboratory technician with a three-dimensional reference of the local soft tissue frame during the fabrication of restorations. The application of this system to orthognathic surgical template fabrication is also discussed. The objective is to obtain the essential esthetic qualities of dentofacial harmony in the laboratory and not at the chairside. This system is compared with other methods of communication.

Frequently, restorative cases received by the dentist from the laboratory have errors in important esthetic parameters, such as occlusal plane or midline. When these errors are discovered during the try-in appointment; either modifications must be made at the chairside or the case must be returned to the laboratory for corrections. Repeated firing of porcelain can eventually degrade its quality and compromise the final esthetics. Ultimately, correction of these errors is time-consuming, costly, and a source of frustration to the doctor, technician, and patient. Exquisite porcelain and masterfully executed crown anatomy cannot compensate for a skewed alignment of the dentogingival complex to the facial planes (Fig. 1).

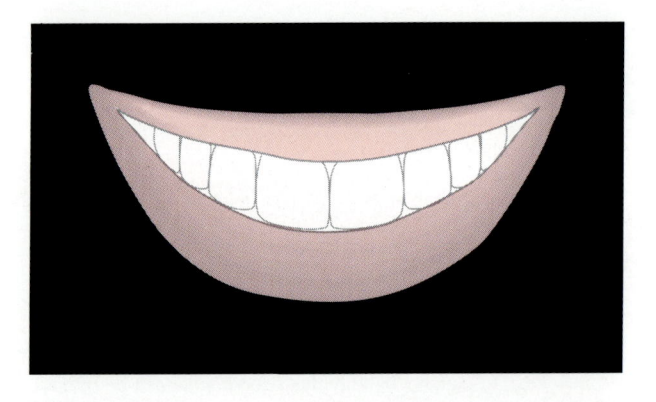

Fig. 2. Smile diagram in which the incisal edges of the maxillary teeth are parallel to the lower lip curvature. (*Modified from* Rifkin and Materdomini [9•].)

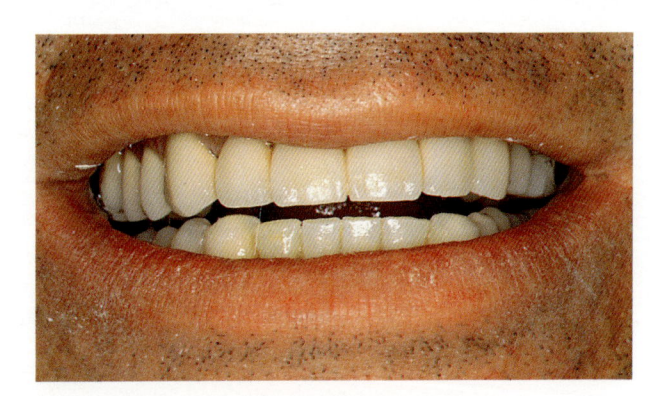

Fig. 1. Unattractive smile alignment.

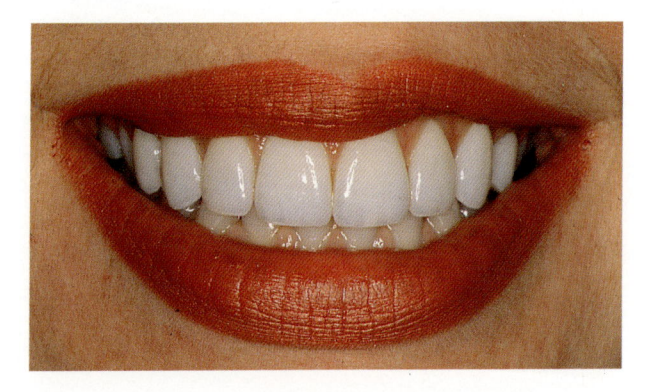

Fig. 3. Attractive smile in facial harmony.

The dental literature is replete with support of the dentolabial relationship and the resultant smile line harmony. Numerous authors agree that the essential elements of an attractive smile are the coinciding of the dental and facial midlines, a level occlusal plane, and a positive incisal smile line that is nearly parallel to the curvature of the upper border of the lower lip [1–7,8•] (Figs. 2 and 3).

Dentofacial references

The lips

The lips are the most important esthetic facial reference in the evaluation of the dental-gingival composition. Artistically, the lips are the "proscenium" of the dentogingival display. They are the most proximal structures to the dentogingival complex by which size, proportion, level, and curvature are visually compared. Because of its proximity, the upper lip has greater visual influence on the maxillary gingival plane; the superior border of the lower lip relates to the maxillary incisal edges and their collective curvature. In space, the lips extend around the face laterally. They are not two dimensional lipstick marks on paper as they are typically illustrated [9•].

In sculpture, frontal, lateral, three-quarter, and overhead views are continuously consulted to evaluate the three-dimensional harmony of all the elements. Similarly, esthetic dentistry is a three-dimensional art, and like the sculptor, the dentist and technician must use multiple views during the esthetic analysis of a smile and the fabrication of dental restorations.

Functional references
Phonetics is a functional reference used to help determine the maximum, not minimum, incisal edge length of the maxillary anterior teeth. The capability of the patient adapt to varying incisal edge positions is evidenced by continuous age-related wear and soft tissue changes without loss of phonetic competency. Phonetics is therefore, not always a reliable reference for esthetics.

Two-dimensional linear references
The interpupillary line is an important frontal linear reference in evaluating contralateral teeth and their lateral-occlusal plane. Camper's line is another linear guide for the anterior-posterior occlusal plane viewed laterally. These two-dimensional linear references are normally used in removable prosthodontics by the dentist at chairside. Both Camper's line and the interpupillary line are straight-line references and do not provide a curvilinear smile-line reference. Only the lips provide this reference.

In removable prosthodontics, wax rims are easily marked and adjusted to guide the laboratory technician in setting teeth. Denture try-ins are also relatively expedient, as opposed to metal or bisque-bake try-ins. In fixed prosthodontics, less information is provided to the technician about facial harmony. Correction of errors in metal and fired porcelain can waste hours of valuable time.

Three-dimensional fabrication references
Until recently, the dentist and not the laboratory technician had the greatest access to the soft tissue of the patients face when evaluating dental restorations [10]. A lip reproduction system developed by Paolo Bertani, first described in 1991 by Grossi, *et al.* [11], manufactured by the Zhermack (Badia Polesine, Italy), and called the Kalco System [12], provides the laboratory technician with the essential three-dimensional soft tissue references.

Lip reproduction system

Materials and technique
The Kalco System materials for lip reproduction include a plastic or metal occlusal tray, a plastic lip impression tray, a large alginate syringe, a variable set nonreversible alginate material for the facial impression, and an addition-reaction silicone putty as the lip replica material (Fig. 4).

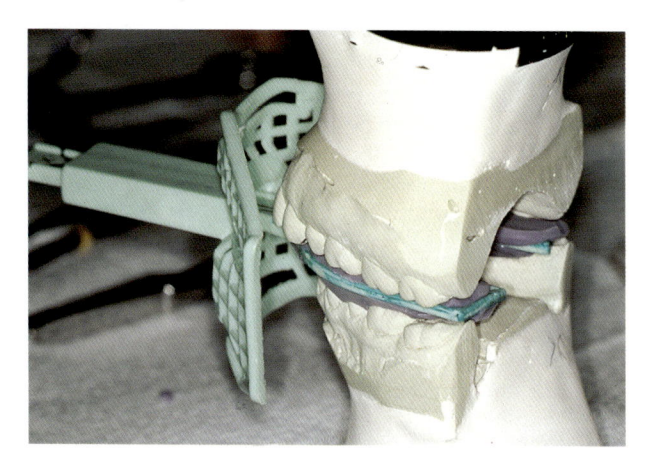

Fig. 4. The Kalco System impression assembly (Zhermack, Badia Polesine, Italy).

The function of the occlusal tray is to transfer the facial impression tray to the dental arches and stabilize it to position the lip replica accurately for the laboratory models. This tray design is one of the most important features of the system.

For fixed prosthodontics, the plastic occlusal tray is fitted to the patient's dental arches and relined with a silicone putty for stabilization in centric relation. This tray has a handle designed to receive the facial impression tray, which slides over the handle and retains the alginate impression material for the actual lip impression.

For removable prosthodontics, the metal occlusal tray is used. This tray is mounted to the maxillary wax bite rim prior to taking the facial impression. The metal is attached to the wax simply by heating it and luting it to the rim. The remainder of the process is identical to that for fixed prosthodontics.

Facial impression and clinical procedures
During the tooth preparation appointment, the facial impression is performed prior to local anesthesia and restorative treatment to avoid impairing lip motor function, which would distort the facial impression. The facial impression begins by fitting the occlusal impression tray to the dental arches (Fig. 5).

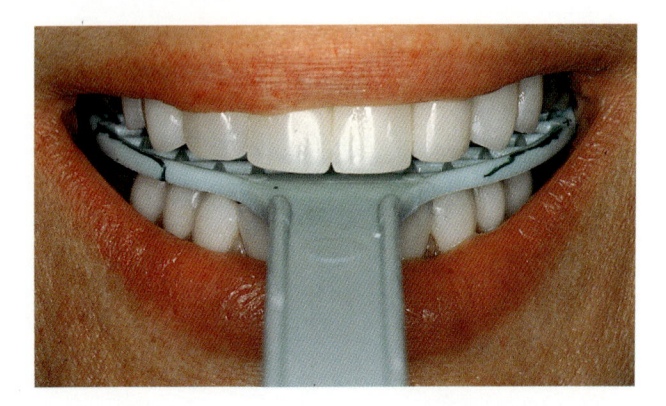

Fig. 5. Occlusal tray position in mouth.

To keep the smile impression as natural as possible, it is important to minimize the occlusal opening during the facial impression and not to have the occlusal tray touch soft facial tissue. This may be accomplished by shortening the length of the occlusal tray and by trimming the width with an acrylic bur. The occlusal tray is then indexed and stabilized on the patient's teeth with a putty or silicone reline material by having the patient close in centric relation. This allows the tray to be mounted between the articulated casts in an accurate and stable position.

The registration should not to be considered an accurate bite registration for occlusion purposes [13]; owing to the intricate variables of hinge axis location, the facebow transfer method, and the degree of vertical opening during the bite registration, the occlusal tray opens the vertical dimension. An actual bite registration should be taken following tooth preparations at the most closed, nondeflected, centric relation position.

Next, slide the facial impression tray over the occlusal tray to within 2 to 4 mm of the face. This distance provides adequate space for the alginate material and prevents any soft tissue distortion by the facial impression tray. This position is marked along the occlusal tray handle for the ensuing impression and later during replica fabrication (Fig. 6). It is imperative that a natural smile be rehearsed by the patient and held for at least 3 minutes while the alginate impression is setting.

The impression is taken by injecting the mixed alginate impression material over the teeth and lips with a syringe and then sliding the alginate loaded tray over the occlusal tray handle, stopping at the predetermined control mark. The alginate setting time can be varied by using the liquid retarder included with the kit. Setting time is approximately 4 to 6 minutes. The patient must now focus on the rehearsed smile and should not be distracted during the impression setting to avoid distorting the smile. Once set, the alginate impression is removed and inspected for accuracy. The facial impression and occlusal tray complex are then stored in a humidor for lip replica fabrication (Fig. 7).

Restorative treatment procedures

After the facial impression is taken, local anesthesia can be administered. Dental preparations, impressions, bite records, facebow transfer, and provisionalization of the prepared teeth are then performed as usual. In one particular case, eight porcelain veneers were used to improve this patient's smile.

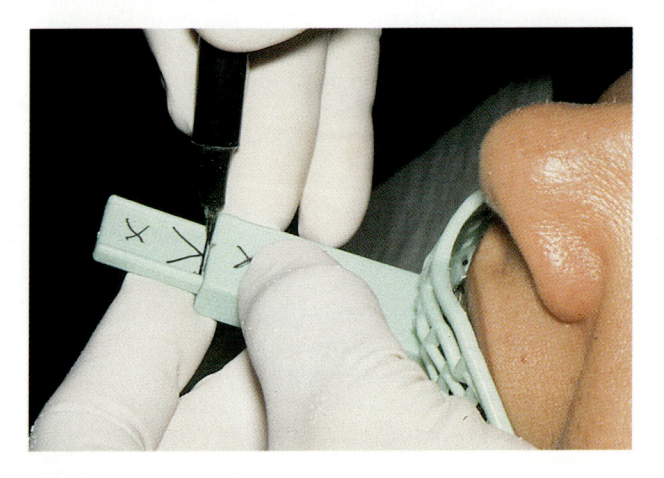

Fig. 6. Space control mark on tray assembly.

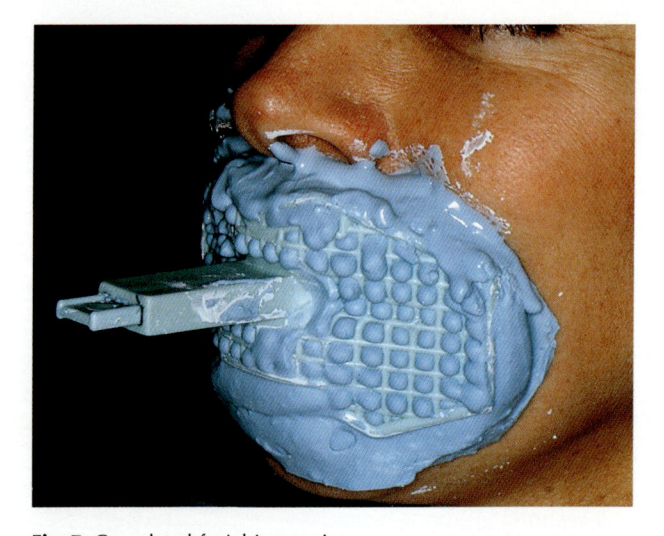

Fig. 7. Completed facial impression.

Facebow transfer
A facially generated facebow technique is highly recommended to mount both diagnostic and working dental casts, especially when the lip reproduction system is not used. The facebow is oriented to the patient's vertical midline and horizontal facial planes.

In addition to the functional benefits of a facebow transfer, the modified facebow transfer technique allows the articulator frame to serve as a reference for the patient's horizontal facial plane and vertical facial midline (Kois and Spear, CRE Lecture, Seattle, 1992) (Figs. 8 and 9).

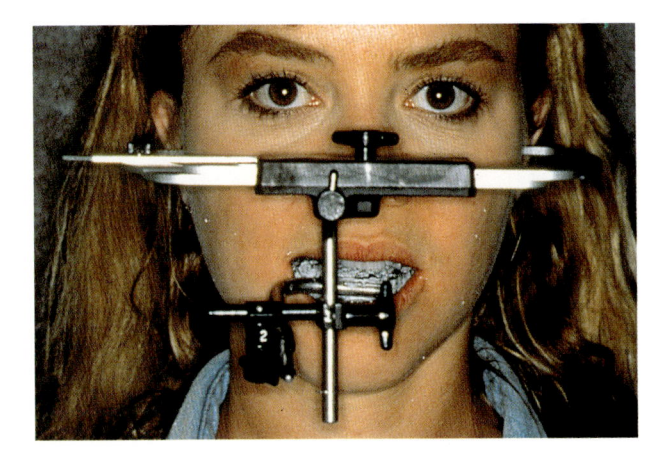

Fig. 8. Facebow with facial midline and horizontal orientation. (*From* Rifkin and Materdomini [9•]; with permission.)

Parallel ruler
A parallel ruler (a marine navigation device not included in the Kalco System) can help to align the facebow with the patient's bipupillary or intercanthus line. It is easier to use the nonmoving intercanthus line rather than track the pupils. The parallel ruler is set on the horizontal arm of the facebow and then expanded to permit the upper half of the ruler to be collinear to the patient's bipupillary line. The horizontal orientation of the facebow is adjusted to be parallel to the patient's bipupillary line. The center of the facebow is also aligned to the patient's facial midline, which may not coincide with the patient's dental midline. The laboratory may now mount the maxillary and mandibular casts and fabricate the facial reproduction.

Laboratory procedures
Once the dental preparation impressions have been poured and the resultant models have been pinned and mounted, the silicone replica of the patient's lips is now created using the alginate facial impression. The mounting stone should be applied smoothly and without undercuts to obtain a retentive yet removable fit for the lip replica. Fabrication time is approximately 30 minutes.

Removal of the incisal pin and platform from the articulator is necessary because they will interfere with the placement of the occlusal tray handle and facial impression. The occlusal impression tray is then placed between the upper and lower mounted models as indexed in the patients mouth.

To confirm accurate seating slide, the facial impression tray onto the occlusal tray, toward the articulated models, until it stops. When necessary, trim the bottom portion of alginate to prevent it from binding to the articulator. Stopping at the indicated control mark provides the accurate thickness of the lips relative to the teeth.

Once complete seating of the facial impression is confirmed, remove it and prepare to create the silicone lip replica. Placing a very thin layer of petroleum jelly lubricant over the models prevents the silicone from sticking to the stone models. The next step is to mix and position the silicone putty within the facial impression and seat it to the prepositioned occlusal tray. Once the putty is thoroughly mixed, incrementally place small strips or pieces of it into the deepest parts of the impression. This will minimize voids and ensure maximum detail.

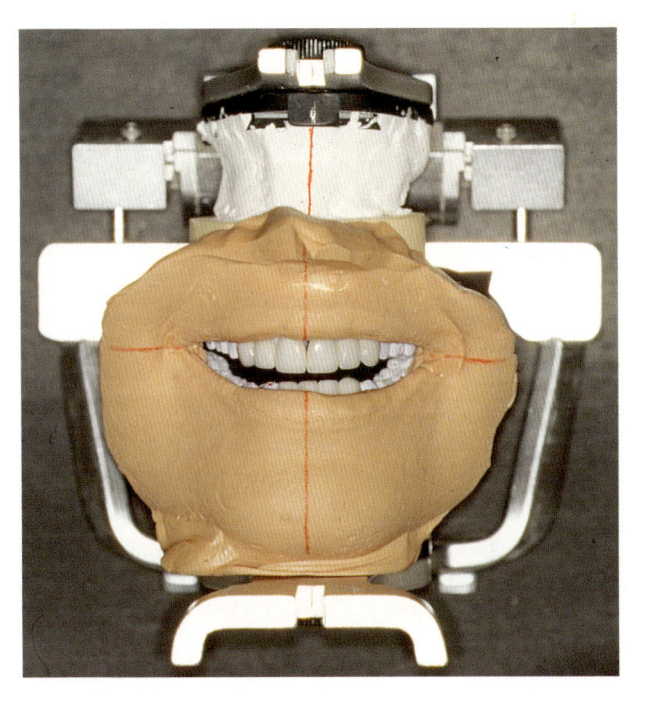

Fig. 9. Mounted case and lip reproduction line references.

Fill the rest of the impression with the remaining material and slide the silicone loaded impression on the positioned occlusal tray handle, stopping at the control mark which confirms complete seating. The silicone will take approximately 15 to 20 minutes to set completely (Fig. 10). Once the silicone material is set, the impression can be removed from the mounted casts.

Remove the excess material from between the lips, using a Bard-Parker knife. Be careful not to cut any part of the lips. Try the lip replica on the model for fit. If any of the silicone prevents complete seating, remove it. Once the models, dies, and lip replica are completed, fabrication of the restorations can proceed.

Restoration fabrication
During fabrication, the ceramist continuously refers to the smile line of the lower lip, the labial midline, and

the commissure line. Individual and collective tooth proportions, alignment, and arrangement are easily visualized and evaluated.

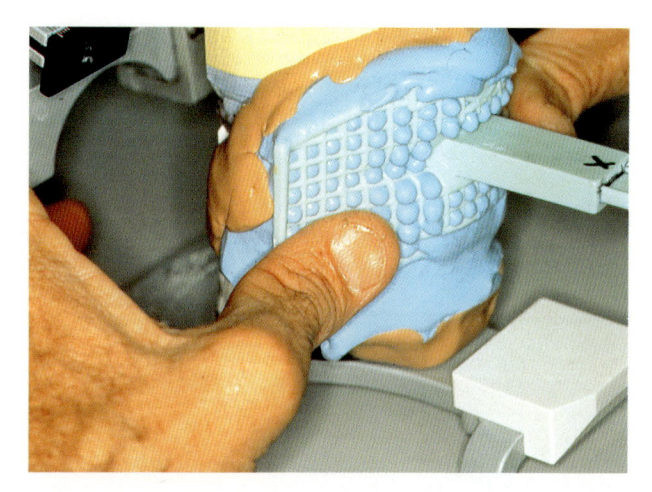

Fig. 10. Seating facial silicone between impression and mounted casts. (*From* Rifkin and Materdomini [9•]; with permission.)

With the lips in place the ceramist can now check the following specific esthetic parameters (Figs. 11 and 12):

1. Midline. With the lips as a centering and vertical reference, it is easy to determine if the restorations follow the facial midline in position and inclination.

2. Smile line. The ceramist can easily follow the curvature of the lower lip of the replica to create a positive dental smile line.

3. Incisal length. Ideally, the dentist should provide the ceramist with dimensions of the teeth, describing their ideal length and width. Dimensional criteria may be based on individual esthetic tooth proportions, phonetics, and considerations such as the patient's preferences, age, race, gender, and upper lip length [14]. With a lip replica, we have an additional reference to evaluate incisal length and curvature.

4. Dentolabial proportional harmony. With the lip replica in place, a proportional harmony between tooth size and lip fullness can be evaluated. Larger teeth may look out of balance and less attractive if the patients lips are thin. In contrast, full lips may permit larger teeth while maintaining proportional harmony.

5. Emergence profile and labial inclination. When the lip replica is viewed laterally, the emergence profile or the labial inclination can be evaluated for lip support and light reflection [8•] (Fig. 13).

6. Internal characterizations. Building dental form and dimension with a three-dimensional reference enables the dental technician to position the porcelain more precisely, reducing the risk of future removal from reshaping. When clinical modifications are minimized, any special effects and characterizations can usually be maintained.

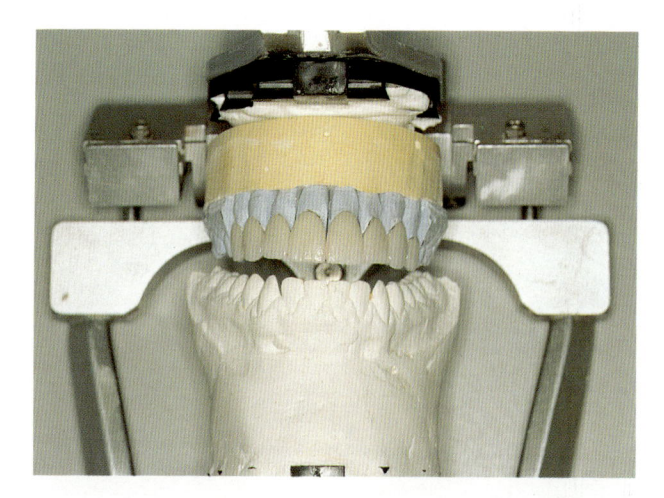

Fig. 11. Porcelain restorations on mounted casts without facial references.

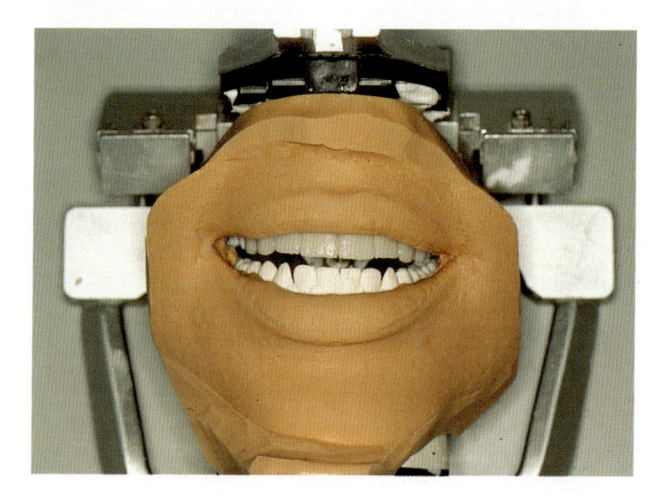

Fig. 12. Frontal view of lip reproduction and restorations during fabrication. (*From* Rifkin and Materdomini [9•]; with permission.)

Cementation

During the appointment for cementation, evaluation of all esthetic parameters and goals is performed prior to the luting of the restorations. If the clinical, facial reproduction and laboratory procedures were accurate, the need for modifications will be minimal and time will be saved by both the dentist and laboratory technician (Fig. 14).

Other esthetic references

Putty core index

Diagnostic or working laboratory models alone seldom provide enough data to assess the smile line reference. A silicone putty labial index taken from a preexisting ideal dentition or a perfected provisional restoration can give the technician three-dimensional esthetic data for direct fabrication [15]. This method requires that the smile line be established and copied. It can be an excellent method and guide for the technician in many situations, but it is not always useful when porcelain veneers are selected, because an accepted dental composition does not yet exist. In these restorative cases, a lip replica is very helpful.

Photographs
Preoperative photographs are useful only as a style design guide for the technician. Photographs are not directly measurable, nor do they serve as a direct working reference.

Computer imaging
Computer imaging is a rapid design tool and an excellent visual communicator for the patient. Like photography, it is limited to conceptual, two-dimensional information, and it does not provide a measurable reference for fabrication in the laboratory (Table 1).

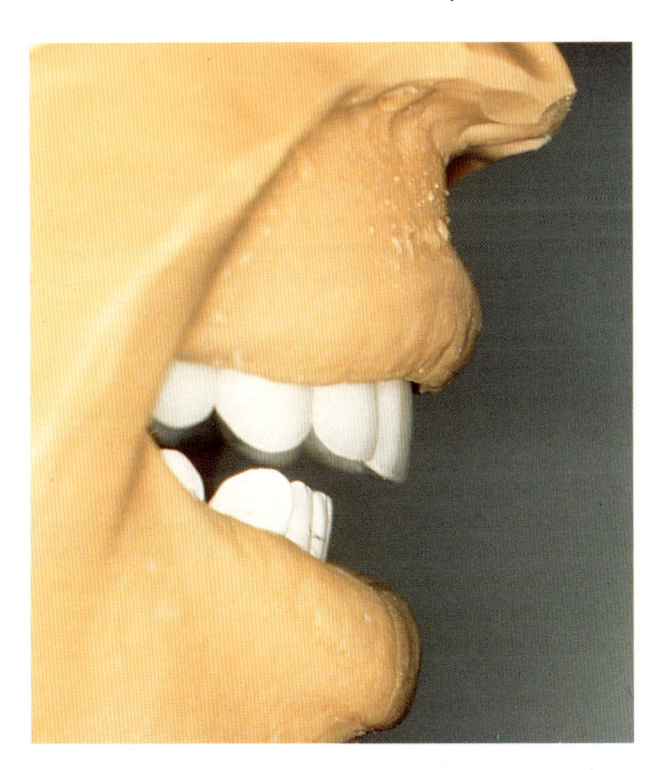

Fig. 13. Lateral view of lip reproduction and restoration inclination. (*From* Rifkin and Materdomini [9•]; with permission.)

Discussion

The advantages experienced in this case presentation and others were in the expeditious, laboratory-established harmony of tooth form, incisal edge position, and smile line. Importantly, no time was required to reshape the incisal edges, and there was no need to return the restorations to the laboratory for rebaking. Thus, intricate incisal edge characterization was preserved, and degradation from multiple refiring of the porcelain was eliminated. Often, in the reshaping of incisal edges, subtle characterizations of the porcelain are lost. Thus, translucency, crack lines, color variation, and the texture so critical to a natural appearance are compromised. Despite the additional time needed to learn this system, with practice, 15 minutes or less is needed for a predictable impression, and less than 30 minutes of laboratory time is needed for the silicone lip fabrication. The time spent in creating a facial reproduction may save considerably more clinical and laboratory time that would be spent correcting basic esthetic errors, thereby reducing the stress involved with chairside try-ins, remakes, and patient disappointment.

Indications and contraindications

The lip reproduction technique should be considered when midline, smile line, and incisal edge position data are either absent or unreliable. It is useful for the following purposes:

1. Fabrication of tooth- or implant-supported single restorations of more than four maxillary anterior teeth

2. Fabrication maxillary anterior fixed partial dentures of three or more teeth involving the midline

3. Incisal lengthening

4. Diastema closure of multiple anterior teeth

5. Long-term anterior provisional restorations

6. Denture fabrication

7. Full mouth or anterior diagnostic wax-up guidance

8. Orthodontic treatment planning

9. Orthognathic maxillary surgical treatment planning and intermaxillary surgical template fabrication for Le Fort osteotomies

Patients exhibiting severely asymmetric smiles, flaccid lips due to poor tissue tones from age or previous multiple collagen or lipid injections, or any difficulty in holding a smile for 3 minutes may be poor candidates for this procedure, because the accuracy of the impression may be diminished.

Orthognathic surgical planning

In orthognathic surgical procedures, consideration must be given to occlusal plane alignment for both

86 Cosmetic dentistry

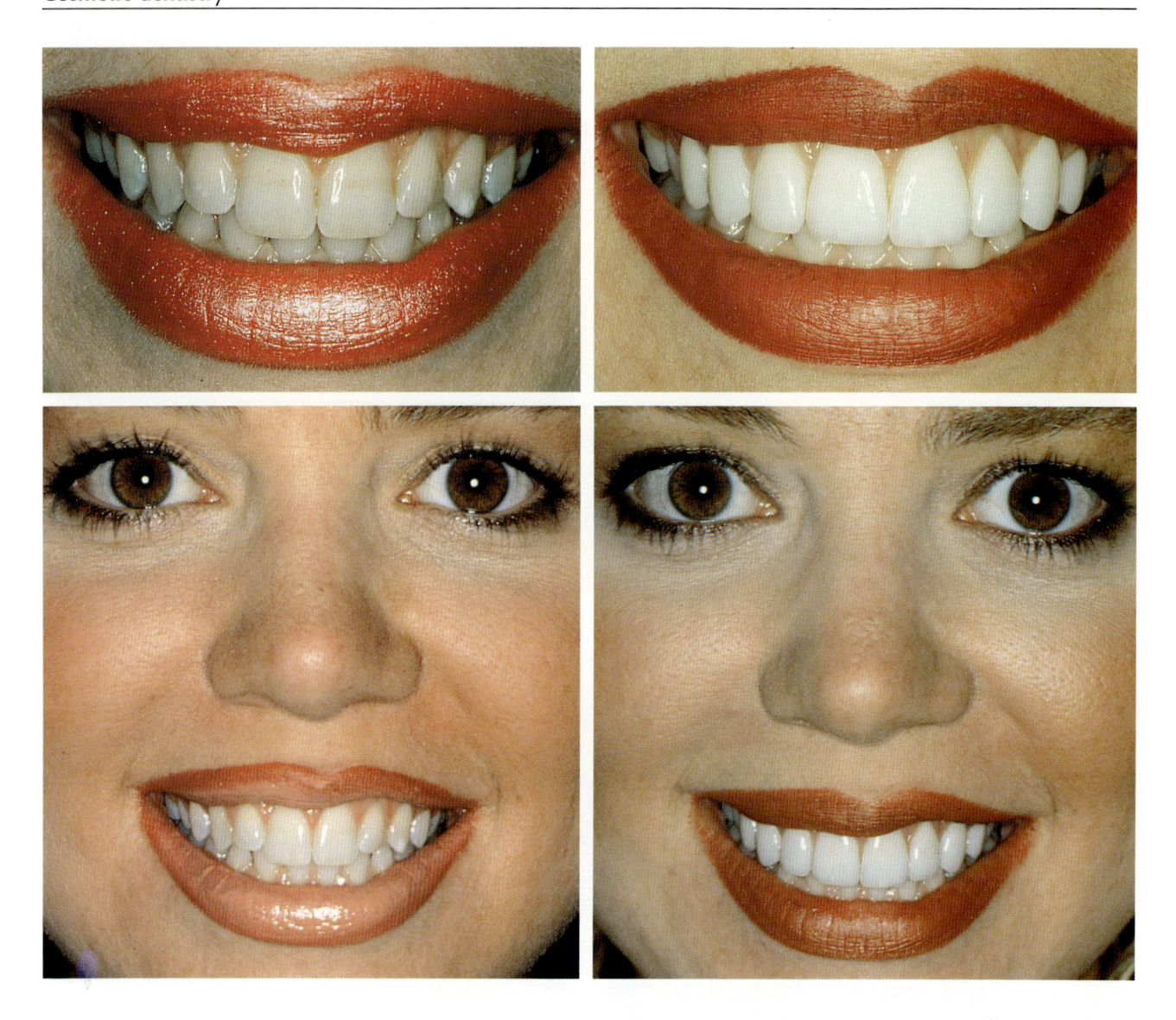

Fig. 14. Top left, Patient's smile before treatment. **Top right,** Patient's smile after placement of eight porcelain restorations. **Bottom left,** Before treatment, full face. **Bottom right,** After treatment. (*From* Rifkin and Materdomini [9•]; with permission.)

Table 1. Comparison of esthetic references for dental restorations		
Reference	Dimensions	Application
Lip reproduction	3	Design and fabrication
Provisional restoration	3	Design and fabrication
Putty core	3	Fabrication
Computer image	2	Design
Photograph	2	Design

functional and esthetic reasons. Consider the treatment planning for a maxillary impaction via the Le Fort surgical procedure [16]. Cephalometrics and computer-assisted measurements have limited accuracy in transferring three-dimensional information to the dental articulator for surgical template fabrication during model surgery (Fig. 15). The accuracy of the template is critical to the positioning and fixation of the maxilla and resultant facial esthetics.

In our case study, the lip reproduction system was used to provide a three-dimensional visual reference during fabrication of an intermaxillary surgical template, which repositioned the separated maxilla and rigidly fixed it to the skull. The final position was thus in harmony with the facial planes (Fig. 16).

The objective was to position accurately and esthetically the surgically separated maxilla with the facially generated template. Thus, the final position of the incisal edge and occlusal plane were in facial-labial harmony at the time of surgery and did not require postsurgical orthodontic correction. During surgery, the facially guided template was used to position the maxilla; bone cut site margins were modi-

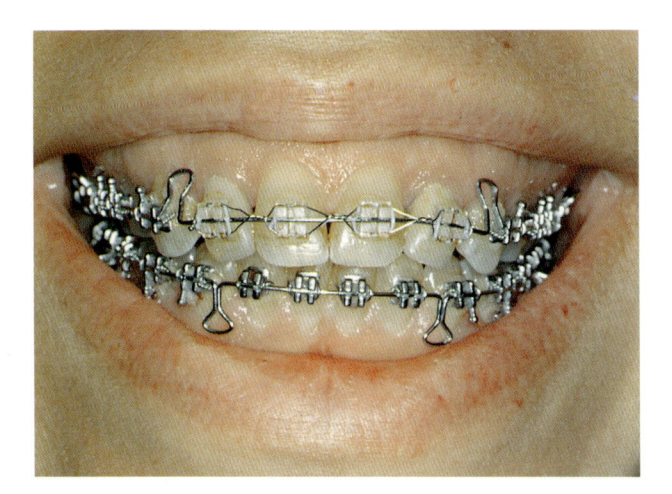

Fig. 15. Presurgical view of vertical maxillary excess.

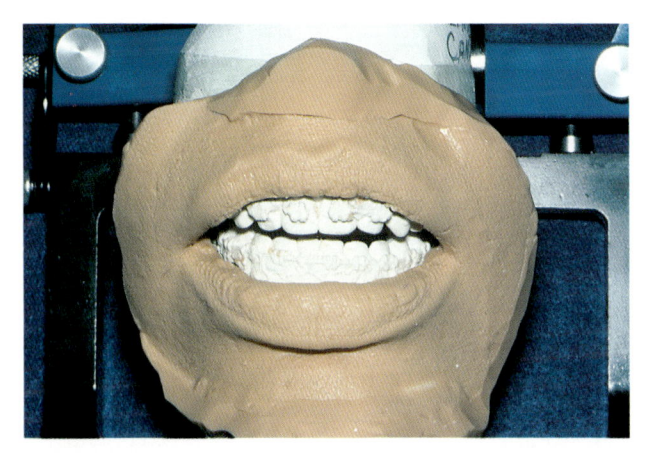

Fig. 16. Lip reproduction reference used during fabrication of an intermaxillary surgical template.

fied for optimal fit, then rigidly fixed for healing (Fig. 17).

At this time, the use of soft tissue references was unpredictable because the soft tissues became flaccid under general anesthesia, and patient was in a supine position. Under such circumstances, an accurately fabricated template rigidly fixed to the mandible may be more reliable (Fig. 18).

The lip reproduction system was not a substitute for comprehensive orthognathic cephalometric and computer-assisted treatment planning. It was used simply as another visual reference.

Recommended improvements

At present, the existing bite-tray is rigid and can increase the vertical dimension a few millimeters beyond normal, resulting in an unnatural smile. Nevertheless, the commissure line, the lower lip curvature, and the midline references may be used as accurate references.

Conclusions

The facial lip reproduction system provides three-dimensional landmarks so that the dental technician may fabricate ceramic restorations more predictably and in harmony with facial structures. When used with other methods, the facial replica adds another dimension to visual references, and once learned, this relatively simple technique can save the dentist, laboratory technician, and patient valuable time and achieve the optimal esthetic result with less stress.

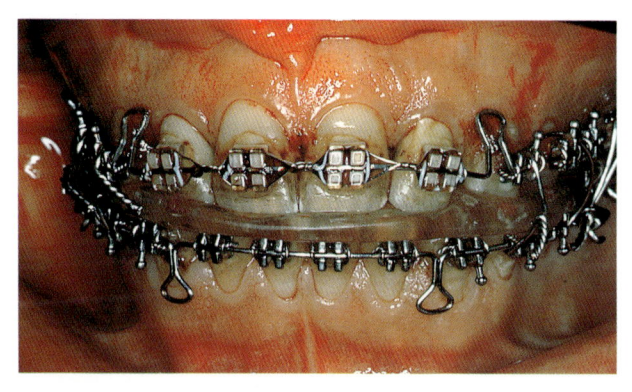

Fig. 17. Intermaxillary surgical template is used to position maxilla during fixation.

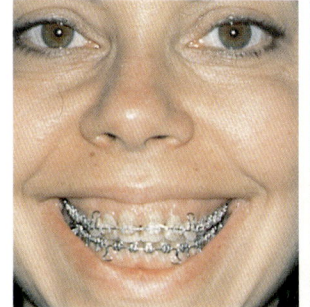

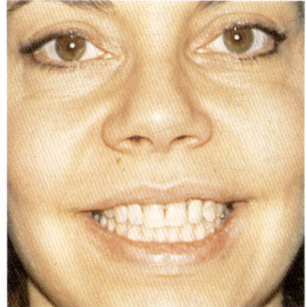

Fig. 18. Left, Before surgery for vertical maxillary excess. **Right,** After surgery, no orthodontics are required to correct facial harmony.

Disclosure

I wish to disclose that I have no commercial interest in the system manufactured by Zhermack or any other lip reproduction system.

Acknowledgments

I want to thank Daniel Materdomini for the laboratory cases presented. Orthodontic treatment was performed by Emanual Wasserman, and orthognathic surgery was performed by Melvyn Wishan, both of whom practice in Beverly Hills, California. Clinical restorative cases were performed by the author.

References and recommended reading

Papers of particular interest, published within the annual period of review, have been highlighted as:
- Of special interest
- •• Of outstanding interest

1. Gysi A: Das Aufstellen einer ganzen Prothese. *Schweiz Monatsschr Zahnheilk* 1915, 25:4.

2. Gysi A: **Unregelmässige Stellung der Frontzähne für prothetische Arbeiten.** *Schweiz Monatsschr Zahnheilk* 1936, 46:58.

3. Goldstein RE: *Esthetics in Dentistry.* Philadelphia: JB Lippincott; 1976.

4. Schulz HH: *Die totale Prothese.* Munich: Neuer Merkur; 1975.

5. Boitel RH: **Aesthetik und Kosmetik in der restaurativen Zahnheilkunde.** *Zahntechnik (Zurich)* 1976, 34:254.

6. Lombardi RE: **The principles of visual perception and their application to denture esthetics.** *J Prosthet Dent* 1973, 29:358–381.

7. Matthews TG: **The anatomy of a smile.** *J Prosthet Dent* 1978, 39:128.

8. Rufenacht CR: *Fundamentals of Esthetics.* Chicago: Quintessence Publishing Co.; 1990.
   Comprehensive textbook of dental esthetics. Includes thorough section on structural esthetic rules, including the components of a smile, lip line, lip variation, and dentolabial composition.

9. Rifkin LR, Materdomini D: **Facial/lip reproduction system for anterior restorations.** *J Esthet Dent* 1993, 5:126–131.
   Demonstrates use of a lip reproduction system for laboratory fabrication of porcelain veneers.

10. Scharer P, Rinn L, Kopp F: *Esthetic Guidelines for Restorative Dentistry.* Chicago: Quintessence Publishing Co.; 1982.

11. Grossi L, Azzalin D, Chiodine M, Bertani P: L'impronta dell'area del sorriso, nuova metodica. *Quintessence Int* 1991, 22:511–514.

12. Bertani P: *Kalco System for Lip Reproduction.* Badia Polesine, Italy: Zhermack.

13. Bertani P: **Sistema per la duplicazione delle labbra relativamente ai denti.** *Estetica* 1992, No. 4:783.

14. Vig RG, Brundo GC: **The kinetics of anterior tooth display.** *J Prosthet Dent* 1972, 39:502.

15. Sze-AJ: **Duplication of anterior provisional fixed partial dentures.** *J Prosthet Dent* 1992, 68:220–223.

16. Conover M, Wishan M: **Computer-assisted orthognathic treatment planning.** *J Calif Dent Assoc* 1994, 22:27–31.

Laurence R. Rifkin, DDS, 414 North Camden Drive, Suite 1280, Beverly Hills, CA 90210, USA

Repairing porcelain and ceramic materials

Didier Cauchie, DDS

Belgian Academy of Esthetic Dentistry, Brussels, Belgium

Technologic breakthroughs in bonding and ceramics have given us materials and techniques that are more reliable in the long term. Nevertheless, we may still be confronted with fractured composites or porcelain. For reasons of finance, technology, psychology, or time, we may find it difficult to abandon the restoration and redo the job. We are then confronted with the problem of repairing the esthetic material, either temporarily or permanently. This paper reviews the recently published articles on techniques and materials used in the repair of dental restorations.

How do fractures occur? The question is important because, as the saying goes, once bitten, twice shy. If it was brought about by an occlusal overload, an abnormal function, a bad habit of the patient, the absence of a supporting structure, or the inadequate design or execution of the restorations, the fracture is obviously bound to recur. It is therefore paramount to identify the mistakes made at the outset. An examination of the fracture will reveal the weak spots in the construction and allow us to draw interesting conclusions about the reconstruction to follow (Fig. 1).

Types of opposing surfaces

The exposed part of the mouth may consist of dentin, enamel, ceramics, metal, composite, or any combination thereof. The repair work may include composite (with an opaque layer, if necessary), porcelain, metal, or a combination of these materials. It is therefore important first of all to examine the possibilities of bonding to these materials individually and then to devise techniques for bonding to them in combination.

Dental tissues

I would be digressing if I described the techniques for bonding to dentin and enamel. Let us simply remember that nowadays, we can achieve bonding strengths greater than the internal cohesive strength of dentin.

Porcelain

Like enamel, porcelain should be etched, although it requires a stronger acid, namely hydrofluoric acid, which creates very small mechanical retention. Wolf et al. [1•] varied the etching time with a 9.5% hydrofluoric acid gel. The highest bonding strength (27 MPa) was obtained with an etching time of 150 seconds. Porcelain simply sanded with aluminum oxide (50 μm) attained a strength of 19 MPa.

Another study showed best results when the porcelain was mechanically roughened with a diamond-charged drill and chemically treated with hydrofluoric acid. Suliman et al. [2••] tested Amalgambond (Parkell Products, Farmingdale, NY), All-Bond 2 enamel bond (Bisco, Itasca, IL), and Clearfil Porcelain Bond (Kuraray Co., Tokyo), on samples of silanated porcelain treated in one of four ways: diamond-roughened, etched with 9.6% hydrofluoric acid gel, sanded for 15 seconds, and diamond-roughened and then acid-etched. The best bonding quality was observed with diamond roughened Clearfil, followed by diamond-roughened, acid etched Amalgambond and diamond-roughened, acid-etched Clearfil. Lu et al. [3] examined bonding to porcelain that was etched, silane-treated, or both; the last category was the most satisfactory.

Appeldoorn et al. [4••] compared repair systems according to their directions for use. After 3 months of water storage and thermocycling, Clearfil Porcelain Bond attained a a shear bond strength of 20.7 MPA, Etch-Free (Parkell Products) a strength of 18.4 MPa, and All-Bond 2 a strength of 17 MPa. In the case of Clearfil, all fractures were cohesive.

In a study of six repair systems, the bonding strengths of five (ranging between 17 and 18.5 MPa) exceeded the cohesive strength of porcelain: All-Bond 2, Clearfil, Metabond (Parkell Products), Scotchprime (3M Dental Products, St. Paul, MN), and Ultradent (Ultradent Products, Salt Lake City, UT) [5]. (These systems do not include all of the required materials; the clinician may use materials of his or her own choosing. In the study, manufacturers' recommendations regarding secondary materials were used for some of the systems.)

Williamson et al. [6] studied the effect of fatigue (with peak stresses of only 2.3 MPa) on the shear bond strength of a resin bonded to porcelain. They found cohesive fractures, from which they concluded that fatigue does not reduce bonding strength. In a study of the fatigue life of repaired (ie, sanded) porcelain, different combinations of composite and repair systems were subjected to longer stress cycles (peak stress = 10.3 MPa) [7•]. Only two, Clearfil Porcelain Bond used in combination with Herculite (Kerr Manufacturing Co., Romulus, MI), and All-Bond (applied with hydrofluo-

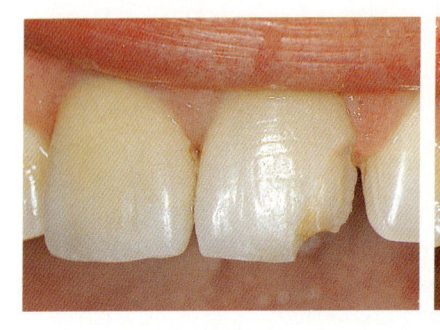

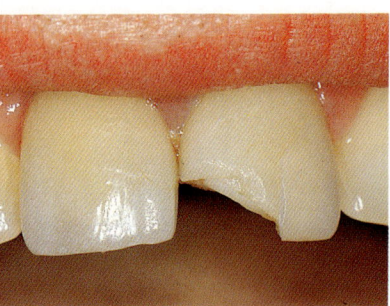

Fig. 1. Left, Fracture of a porcelain laminate veneer. **Right,** After placement of a temporary repair, a second fracture occurred, but in a different place. The repair seemed stronger than the original bond. (*Courtesy of* P. Kroff, Brussels, Belgium.)

ric acid, porcelain primer, and dentin-enamel bonding resin) used in combination with Bisfil (Bisco), survived 2 million stress cycles. It is worth noting that the same adhesives failed when they were combined with microfill composites under very small stresses.

We can reasonably conclude that Clearfil Porcelain Bond offers an easy and reliable system; it is sufficient to roughen with sanding or a diamond-charged drill before the mixture is applied. In an alternative system, the porcelain is sanded, etched with hydrofluoric acid, and treated with silane before the bonding resin is applied. In this case, the All-Bond and Scotchprime kits have proved their effectiveness.

Composite

The first question we have to ask ourselves is whether the repair of aged composites requires etching with hydrofluoric acid. Swift *et al.* [8] attempted to evaluate the effects of sanding, etching, silane treatment, and a combination of these procedures on the bonding to a hybrid composite, namely Herculite. After thermocycling, the best bonding quality (28.4 MPa) with the smallest standard deviation (3.7 MPa) was found in air-abraded, silane-treated composite, which far outperformed etched composite. A second study of different makes and types of composite showed that although the bond strength of certain composites may be increased with hydrofluoric acid etching, this increase is not significant [9]. It also showed that hydrofluoric acid can impair the bonding strength of certain composites. Because very often we do not know the composition of the composite to be repaired, sanding is recommended. These findings were confirmed in a study of bond strength of a resin cement to a hybrid inlay composite (Triad; Dentsply International, York, PA) [10••]. The best preparation of a polymer composite consisted of abrasion with aluminum oxide, 50 µm, followed by the application of a layer of bonding resin. The figures for shear bond strength were on the same order as those for the bonding of resin cement to enamel (etched with phosphoric acid). Neither hydrofluoric acid nor aluminum bifluoride could guarantee solid bonding to composite.

A study of indirect composites in bracket bonding in orthodontia examined the interface of sealants and aged composites [11]. Although the study was irrelevant in terms of the products and techniques used, it is nevertheless interesting to note that the best bonding quality was obtained when the polymerized composite had been treated with acetone. On the other hand, Turner *et al.* [12•] established that the surface roughness has a greater effect than the bonding agent, and that the All-Bond system gives the best bonding result. As a matter of fact, the A and B primers of All-Bond use acetone as a solvent. Is this the reason for their performance, viscosity, and wettability? In any event, Concept resin (Ivoclar-Williams, Amherst, NY) repaired with Heliomolar (Ivoclar-Vivadent, Amherst, NY) resisted fracturing better when it had been air-abraded rather than sanded and when the All-Bond system was used, rather than Special Bond 2 (Ivoclar-Vivadent) or Heliobond (Ivoclar-Vivadent).

For obvious reasons of toxicity, it is reassuring to be able to avoid using hydrofluoric acid for repairing composite. Although we may be confronted with different kinds of composite stress and variable physicochemical properties, it clearly seems a good idea of prepare the composite surface by sanding it with aluminum oxide, 50 µm, and then applying a bonding resin. Between these two stages, the application of a highly hydrophilic primer such as All-Bond A or B is likely to improve the bonding quality.

Composite and tooth

Such a combination, frequent in cases of fracture, poses no problem. After the residual bonding agent is drilled away from the enamel or dentin, the technique described above can be perfectly applied: sanding, hydrofluoric acid etching, and application of All-Bond 2 primer and bonding resin. The only additional challenge might be the etching of the dental tissues with phosphoric acid.

Metal and ceramics

We currently know that 1) the bond strengths of the noble and high-noble alloys are significantly greater when they are tin-plated [13]; 2) because of the risk of surface oxidation, it is not advisable to bring hydrofluoric acid into contact with metal (Bertolotti, Paper presented in Brussels, 1992); 3) a layer of opaque composite can be used without reducing the bond strength [14]; and 4) prehydrolized silanes guarantee a better bonding to metal than silanes with two components [15•]. (The best result was obtained with Scotchprime on nickel-chromium.)

The technique for repairing ceramics and metal can therefore proceed as follows:

1. Preparation of the bonding surface with a diamond-charged drill

2. Aluminum oxide sanding of the porcelain and metal

3. Tin-plating of the noble metal, if appropriate

4. Application of Clearfil Porcelain Bond, or application of silane followed by primer [16]

5. Application of opaque composite, composite, or composite cement

Conclusions

Intrabuccal repairs of composite or porcelain have been the final hurdle in bonding dentistry. The techniques and materials currently available are insufficient to guarantee perfect bonding under all circumstances. Nevertheless, certain facts do allow us to increase our chances of success:

The intrabuccal air abrader is an indispensable tool

Silane treatment increases the regularity of success

Low-viscosity hydrophilic primers also seem to help in most cases

Apart from these considerations, all the information currently available with respect to direct (ie, composite) or indirect (ie, composite, ceramic, or ceramic and metal) fillings allows us to choose the ideal material and technique for restorations. As we have seen, the circumstances of the fracture and the reasons we decide to repair rather than replace are so varied that it is impossible to provide for all cases. Caution is in order; all studies indicate a certain failure rate. We are awaiting the results of new research now being carried out *in vivo*. This research will be useful, because it is based on realistic working conditions (taking into account such factors as relative humidity), uses today's materials, and asks the right questions to get the right answers, of which there are today very few.

References and recommended reading

Papers of particular interest, published within the annual period of review, have been highlighted as:
* Of special interest
** Of outstanding interest

1. Wolf DM, Powers JM, O'Keefe KL: **Bond strength of composite to etched and sandblasted porcelain.** *Am J Dent* 1993, 6:155–158.
   •
The authors studied the bonding strength of composite to etched and sanded porcelain. They varied the etching time with a 9.5% hydrofluoric acid gel and obtained the highest bonding strength (27 MPa) with an etching time of 150 seconds. Porcelain simply sanded with aluminum oxide attained a strength of 19 MPa.

2. Suliman AH, Swift EJ Jr, Perdigao J: **Effects of surface treatment and bonding agents on bond strength of composite resin to porcelain.** *J Prosthet Dent* 1993, 70:118–120.
   ••
Suggests that in terms of bonding strength, the bonding system is more important than the method used to treat the surface of the porcelain.

3. Lu R, Harcourt JK, Tyas MJ, Alexander B: **An investigation of the composite resin/porcelain interface.** *Aust Dent J* 1992, 37:12–19.

4. Appeldoorn RE, Wilwerding TM, Barkmeier WW: **Bond strength of composite resin to porcelain with newer generation porcelain repair systems.** *J Prosthet Dent* 1993, 70:6–11.
   ••
Reports on bond strength of composite resin to porcelain and concludes that some new repair systems provide adequate bonding for the long term.

5. Diaz Arnold AM, Wistrom DW, Aquilino SA, Swift EJ Jr: **Bond strengths of porcelain repair adhesive systems.** *Am J Dent* 1993, 6:291–294.

6. Williamson RT, Mitchell RJ, Breeding LC: **The effect of fatigue on the shear bond strength of resin bonded porcelain.** *J Prosthodont* 1993, 2:115–119.

7. Llobell A, Nicholls JL, Kois JC, Daly CH: **Fatigue life of porcelain repair systems.** *Int J Prosthodont* 1992, 3:205–213.
   •
Reports that some repair systems can survive stress if combined with hybrid composites.

8. Swift EJ Jr, Brodeur C, Cvitko E, Pires JAF: **Treatment of composite surface for indirect bonding.** *Dent Mater* 1992, 5:193–196.

9. Swift EJ Jr, Le Valley BD, Boyer DB: **Evaluation of new methods for composite repair.** *Dent Mater* 1992, 11:362–365.

10. Latta MA, Barkmeier WW: **Bond strength of a resin cement to a cured composite inlay material.** *J Prosthet Dent* 1994, 72:189–193.
    ••
Reports findings that sandblasting outperforms hydrofluoric acid etching for hybrid composites.

11. Shiau JY, Rasmussen ST, Phelps AE, Enlow DH, Wolf GR: **Analysis of the "shear" bond strength of pretreated aged composites used in some indirect bonding techniques.** *J Dent Res* 1993, 72:1291–1297.

12. Turner CW, Meiers JC: **Repair of an aged, contaminated indirect composite resin with direct, visible light-cured composite resin.** *Oper Dent* 1993, 18:187–194.
    •
Reports that for Concept inlays, the highest bond strength is produced by air abrasion, followed by All-Bond treatment.

13. Gates W, Diaz-Arnold A, Aquilino S, Ryther J: **Comparison of the adhesive strength of a Bis-GMA cement to tin-plated and non–tin-plated alloys.** *J Prosthet Dent* 1993, 69:12–16.

14. Pagniano RP, Longnecker S: **Shear resistance of composite resin to enamel using color-modifying resins and variously applied unfilled bonding resin.** *J Prosthet Dent* 1991, 4:445–450.

15. Anagnostopoulos T, Eliades G, Palaghias G: **Composition, reactivity and surface interactions of three dental silane primers.** *Dent Mater* 1993, 5:182–190.
    •
Reports on research into surface interaction and bond strength. The authors found that prehydrolized silane provides significant advantages over two-component systems.

16. **Porcelain-fused-to-metal crown repair.** *Clinical Research Associates Newsletter* 1994, 16:3–4.

Didier Cauchie, DDS, 440 avenue Louise, 1050 Brussels, Belgium.

A case study of lasers in cosmetic dentistry

Harvey Passes, DDS,* Morey Furman, DDS,* David Rosenfeld, DDS,* and Adrian Jurim, MDT†

*Jamaica Hospital, Jamaica, New York, and †Jamaica, New York, USA

The dental laser offers revolutionary advantages over traditional cosmetic dental treatment for our patients. These advantages include precision, hemostasis, sterility, and minimal postoperative pain and swelling. The laser interacts with tissue to vaporize it in a predictable manner that produces predictable results. It is used in periodontal plastic surgery, gingivectomy, soft-tissue crown lengthening, crown and bridge gingival retraction, composite curing, biopsy, frenectomy, stage II implant recovery, and more. Fixed prosthetic impressions can be taken immediately following gingivoplasty and sutures and postoperative dressings are eliminated. This paper presents a case study in cosmetic dentistry to demonstrate many of these applications and summarizes current opinion regarding them. It also briefly describes what a laser is and how it works.

What is a laser?

Before describing the revolutionary features, advantages, and benefits the dental laser offers over traditional treatment for our patients, we must explain what a laser is and how it interacts with tissue. The dental laser is an instrument that can vaporize tissue. Its energy is produced by electrically stimulating different elements within a concave mirrored chamber. This concentrated energy is then harnessed and allowed to leave the chamber as a fine stream of photons. Finally, it is directed to the target tissue by an accurate delivery system.

Lasers achieve the desired results by interacting with tissue. The energy created is predictable and dependent on the material that produces it. There are five commercially available dental lasers. They are holmium:yttrium-aluminum-garnet, neodymium:yttrium-aluminum-garnet (Nd:YAG), carbon dioxide (CO_2), argon, and erbium:yttrium-aluminum-garnet.

The laser can interact with tissue in one of four ways: absorption, transmission, reflection, or scatter. For laser energy to be effective, it must be absorbed by the target tissue. This absorption allows the energy to vaporize the tissue and produce the desired result. The dental laser can be applied to any procedure in which tissue needs to be reduced, excised, reshaped, or sealed. Some of these applications include gingivectomy, gingivoplasty, frenectomy, biopsy, distal wedge and tuberosity reduction, hemostasis, crown and bridge and restorative gingival retraction, stage II implant recovery, and composite curing for restorative procedures. There are five primary reasons for replacing traditional treatments with the dental laser: 1) Precision: The dental laser offers unusual accuracy in tissue interaction because of its delivery system and its ability for shallow tissue absorption. 2) Sterility: Microorganisms are killed after exposure to the laser [1]. 3) Minimal postoperative swelling: Lymphatics are sealed at the surgical site [2•]. 4) Minimal postoperative pain [2•–4•]: The nerve endings are also sealed at the surgical site. 5) Hemostasis: Blood loss is minimal owing to sealing of the blood vessels at the surgical site [5••,6], which also offers improved visibility during the surgical procedure. In most instances, postoperative dressings and sutures are not required. All of these features offer advantages to this treatment over the traditional approach. Furthermore, reports have described good patient acceptance of the laser [4•].

After a brief history on the origin and progression of the dental laser, we shall discuss the different dental lasers and their specific applications (Table 1) and then present a case study in which some of these lasers were used to achieve a cosmetic result.

Brief history

The idea of the laser was first conceived by Albert Einstein around the turn of the century. He demonstrated mathematically the possibility that portions of an electromagnetic field could be stimulated to emit amplified light. The term *laser* is an acronym for *light amplification by stimulated emission of radiation*. In 1960, Maiman [7] inserted a ruby rod into a photographic flash lamp to establish the first laser. Since its incep-

---

Abbreviation
Nd:YAG—neodymium:yttrium-aluminum-garnet.

Table 1. Lasers and their clinical applications

Type	Wavelength, nm	Absorption properties	Medium	Advantages	Delivery system
CO_2	10,600	H_2O in tissue	Gas	Gross reduction and rapid vaporization of soft tissue; Good hemostasis	Hollow wave guide; Articulated arm
Neodymium:yttrium-aluminum-garnet	1064	Dark pigmented tissue	Solid	Surgical precision; Excellent hemostasis; Soft-tissue sculpting	Quartz fiber optic
Holmium	2100	H_2O in tissue	Solid	Rapid vaporization of soft tissue; Hard tissue uses, eg, temporomandibular joint surgery	Quartz fiber optic
Argon	476, 488, 514	Hemoglobin	Gas	Rapid evaporation of soft tissue; Hard tissue use; curing composites	Quartz fiber optic with a bare fiber
Erbium	2936	H_2O in tissue; Bone: organic matrix; inorganic matrix; calcium salts	Solid	Rapid evaporation of soft tissue; Potential candidate to replace dental drill	Articulated arm; Fiber optic being developed

tion, lasers have found their way into many fields and applications. In the field of medicine, the laser has replaced the scalpel in the removal of various lesions. Numerous medical specialists use lasers routinely. It is not uncommon to find the argon, the CO_2, or the Nd:YAG laser in the offices of ophthalmologists, gynecologists, dermatologists, and plastic surgeons. The early 1960s witnessed the beginning of the dental research in lasers. Most of the early work explored the effects of lasers on enamel, dentin, and pulpal tissue [8]. As time passed, researchers realized the potential for laser use in other disciplines. The research expanded into endodontics [9,10] and periodontics [11,12]. In the early 1970s, CO_2 lasers became commercially available for medical applications. The CO_2 laser was not practical for use in dentistry until the mid-1980s, when the hollow wave guide delivery system was developed. The development of the fiber optic delivery system paved the way for use of other lasers in dentistry. Clinicians and researchers who use these instruments have developed organizations for research, education, and training, which include the Academy of Laser Dentistry and the International Society of Laser Dentistry.

Types of lasers and clinical applications

CO_2 laser
The CO_2 laser has a wavelength of 10,600 nm. Its active media are carbon dioxide, nitrogen, and helium. All of the CO_2 lasers on the market today are continuous-wave. The CO_2 laser wavelength is strongly absorbed by the water component of tissue. There is a high percentage of water in soft tissue, which allows for its rapid vaporization [13••]. The typical zone of necrosis is approximately 100 μm when soft tissue is cut. The CO_2 laser provides hemostasis and surgical precision. Its wavelength is well suited to the ablation of gross fibrous tissue. Applications include gingivectomy, gingivoplasty, soft-tissue crown lengthening, frenectomy, biopsy, gingival troughing, gingival retraction, and tuberosity reduction [14••,15]. The CO_2 laser's delivery system uses a hollow wave guide or an articulated arm. Various tip sizes are designed for the specific application. For example, smaller tips are used for gingival contouring, and larger ones for gross ablation as in tuberosity reductions.

Neodymium:yttrium-aluminum-garnet laser
Current Nd:YAG dental lasers emit a wavelength of 1064 nm. This laser uses a solid state active medium. The Nd:YAG laser relies on its absorption into dark pigmented tissue for its effectiveness. The quartz fiber optic delivery system gives the dentist great control and flexibility in the operating field. The Nd:YAG laser cuts soft tissue in the contact mode (the fiber is in physical contact with the tissue), whereas the noncontact mode is used for coagulation and hemostasis. Thermal zones of necrosis less than 1 mm can be achieved. Excellent hemostasis and surgical precision for soft-tis-

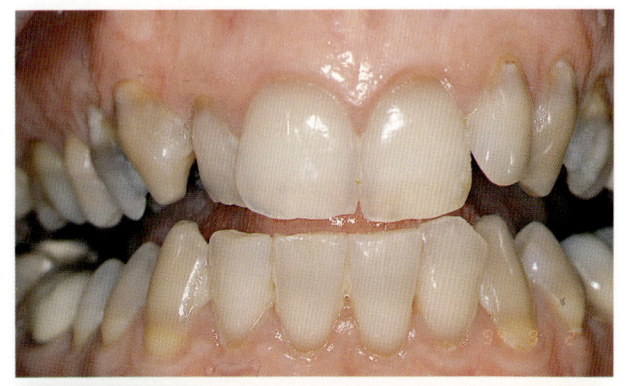

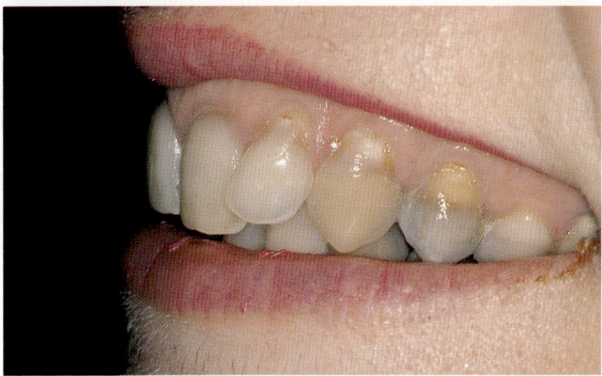

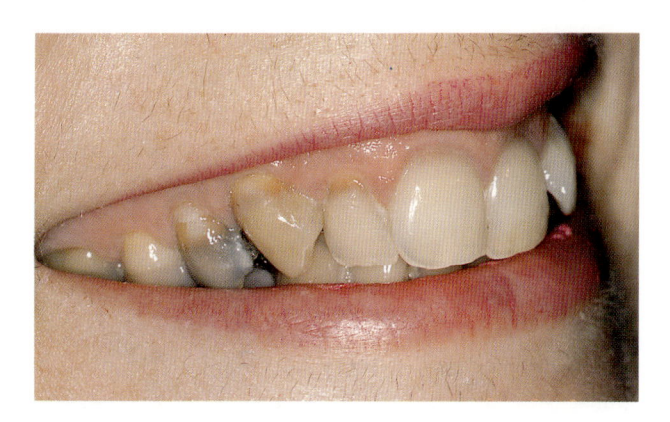

Fig. 1. Preoperative views of a 32-year-old woman who presented herself for cosmetic treatment of her upper anterior teeth. Note irregular gingival contour and severe tetracycline staining.

sue procedures are obtained. Nd:YAG lasers are used for soft-tissue sculpting, as in papillary and irritative fibrosis, gingivoplasty, gingivectomy, gingival troughing, frenectomy; treatment of aphthous and herpetic ulcers; and the sterilization of periodontal pockets [15,16,17•].

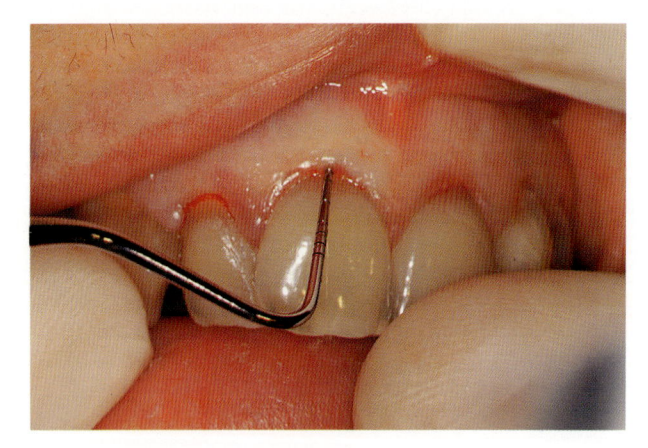

Fig. 2. Periodontal pocket probing.

Holmium laser

The holmium laser is a free-running pulsed laser with a wavelength of 2100 nm. It can cut and vaporize soft tissue, like the CO_2 laser, with the added advantage of a quartz optical fiber delivery system [13••]. A bare optic fiber is used in the contact mode for rapid cutting, and the noncontact mode is used for hemostasis. The hemostasis provided by this laser is more effective than that provided by the CO_2 laser, but less effective than that provided by the Nd:YAG laser. Holmium lasers have the approval of the US Food and Drug Administration for use on hard tissue for temporomandibular joint surgery in which cartilage is reshaped. Hard-tissue applications, such as caries removal, dentin modification, enamel etching, and bone ablation, are currently being explored [18]. The potential exists for this wavelength to cut enamel and dentin. The holmium laser is used in second stage implant recovery and in rapid tissue ablation (Passes *et al.*, Papers presented at the International Academy of Laser Dentistry Second annual Meeting, Honolulu, 1992). The holmium laser beam is strongly absorbed by the water component of tissue.

Argon laser

Argon lasers are continuous-wave lasers. The blue-green wavelengths are emitted in 476, 488, and 514 nm. These wavelengths are absorbed strongly by hemoglobin. This characteristic allows the argon laser to cut, vaporize, and coagulate most types of tissue. The argon laser exhibits good surgical precision and hemostasis; however, the laser's cutting efficiency decreases in hemoglobin-poor tissues [18]. Presently, the argon laser is the only laser cleared by the US Food and Drug Administration for hard-tissue application in dentistry. It is used to cure composites fully and evenly [14••,17•,19,20], which is accomplished under low power. A bare quartz fiber is used for delivering the lower energy to the surgical site. The fiber must be used in contact or near-contact mode to cut and vaporize soft tissue.

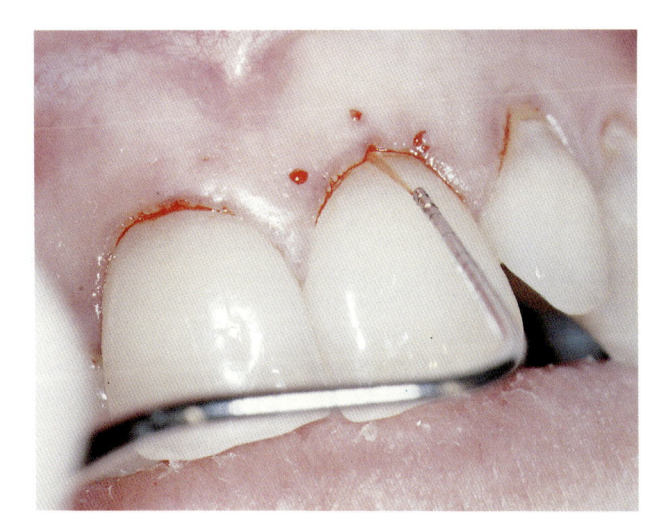

Fig. 3. Periodontal probe bleeding points indicate the extent of the superior position of the finished result.

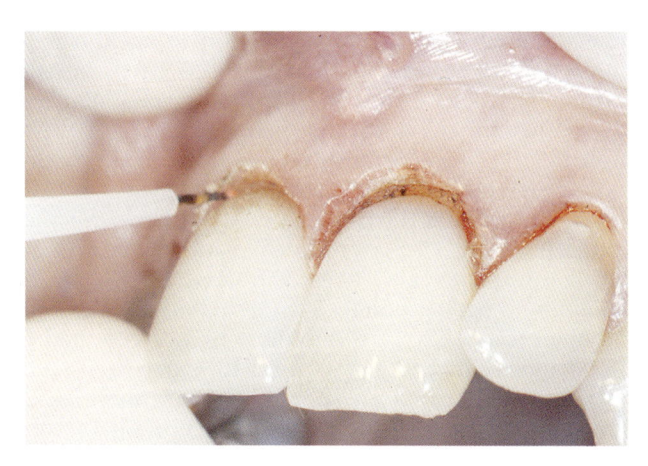

Fig. 4. Tissue sculpting using the free-running neodymium:yttrium-aluminum-garnet laser at 35 Hz and 3.25 W.

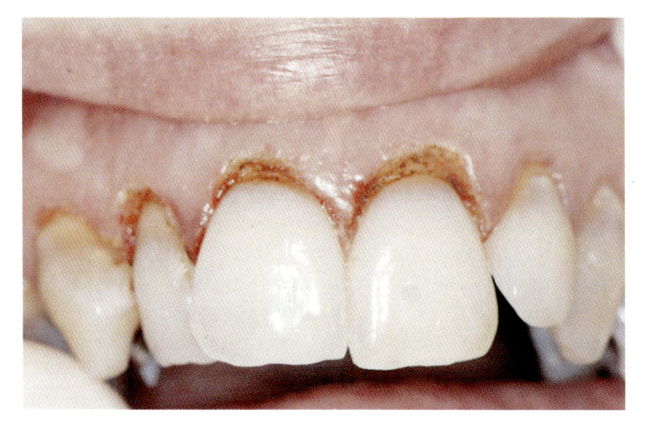

Fig. 5. Immediate postoperative view after tissue sculpting with laser.

Erbium laser

The erbium laser has the ability to cut enamel and dentin and might possibly replace the dental drill for the treatment of dental caries. The erbium wavelength of 2936 nm is absorbed by water, organic matrix, and inorganic calcium salts that comprise bone, enamel, and other hard biologic materials [13••]. The erbium laser has shallow tissue penetration, which allows it to ablate soft tissue with the surgical precision of a scalpel but with poor hemostasis. The currently available delivery system for the erbium laser is an articulated arm. Fiber delivery systems are expected on the US market soon.

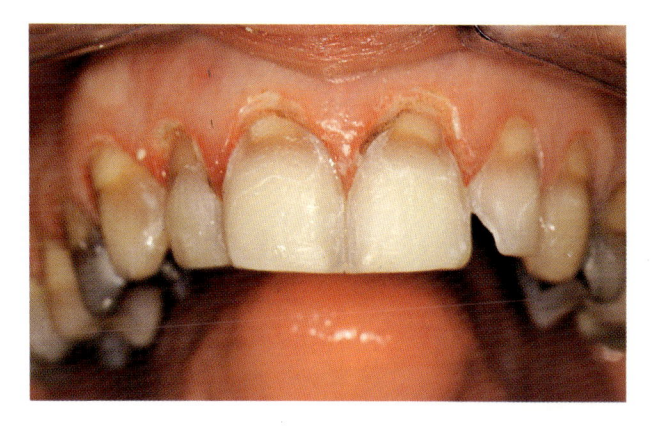

Fig. 6. Veneer preparations completed.

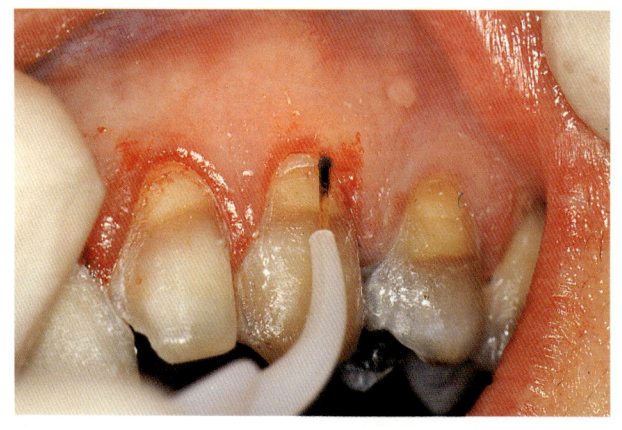

Fig. 7. Sulcular troughing with the neodymium:yttrium-aluminum-garnet laser prior to impression.

Case study

A 32-year-old woman presented herself for cosmetic treatment of her upper anterior teeth. Clinical examination revealed severely misaligned, tetracycline-stained teeth (Fig. 1). She explained that this disfigurement had caused her much embarrassment throughout her life. Previous attempts at bleaching had not relieved her condition. She asked about her options for creating a more esthetic smile. She also brought her uneven gumline to our attention.

Clinical examination demonstrated periodontal pocketing from 3 to 5 mm throughout her periodontium with slight bleeding on probing (Fig. 2). No mobil-

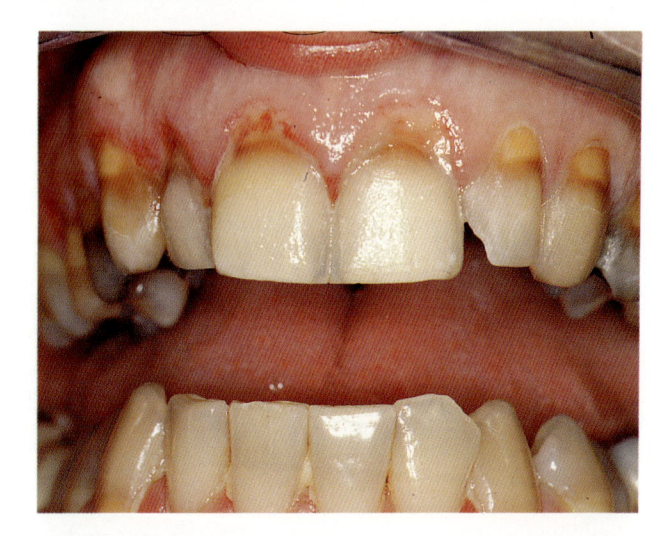

Fig. 8. Postoperative result 2 days after sulcular troughing. Note the appearance of the soft tissue.

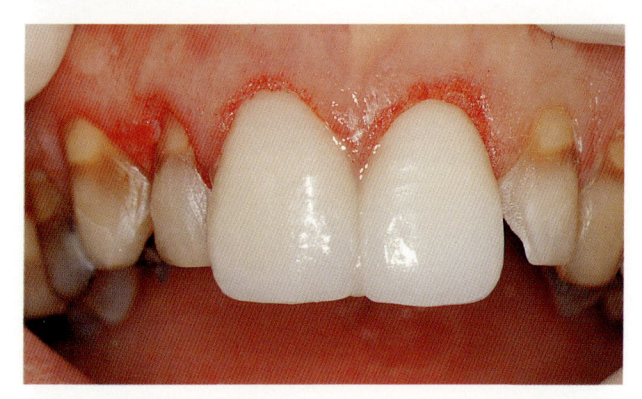

Fig. 9. Porcelain veneer try-in.

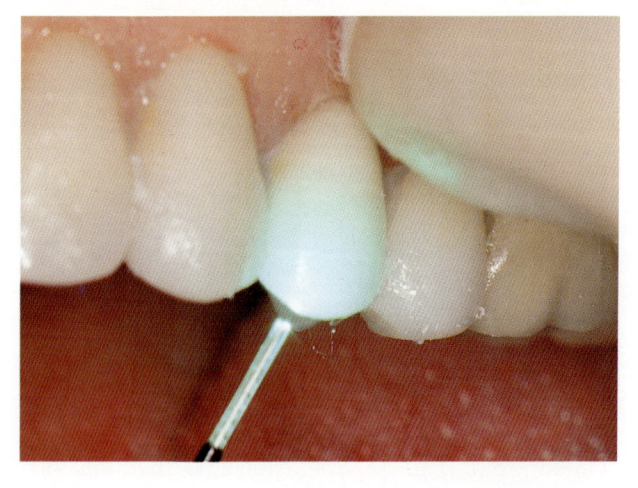

Fig. 10. Curing of porcelain veneer bond with an argon laser.

ity was observed. Radiographs revealed good supportive bone with no evidence of pathology. Tooth vitality appeared to be within normal limits. The most obvious condition was the clinical crowding of her anterior teeth with erratic gingival height. A mild case of gingivitis was diagnosed. After periodontal scaling, root planing, and prophylaxis treatment, it was deter- mined that laser gingivoplasty would be performed, followed by the seating of porcelain laminate veneers. This treatment plan would cosmetically reconstruct her smile line while realigning and brightening her teeth. Treatment would begin with teeth 4 through 13. Her lower teeth would be treated in the future. After the treatment was explained, the patient gave informed consent. There were no contraindications to treatment. The indications for porcelain laminate veneer coverage was based on its expedient conservative restorative nature and its ability to give the patient her desired shade. The indications for laser gingival surgery are discussed in greater detail below.

Treatment sequence

The patient was brought to the operatory, seated, and draped in the usual manner. An infiltration of 108 mg of 2% lidocaine 1:50,000 epinephrine was administered to teeth 4 through 13. Periodontal probe bleeding points were indicated between 2 to 3 mm superiorly to the gingival crest of each tooth except number 11; its height was already at the most superior position for the finished result (Fig. 3). The Excel Technology (Haupage, NY) free-running pulsed Nd:YAG laser was used at 35 Hz and 3.25 W to contour the gingival tissue. The laser energy was delivered with a 300-μm quartz optic fiber. The tissue was sculpted using the bleeding points as a guide (Fig. 4). The optic fiber was gently placed at the gingival crest, and a back and forth motion was used to ablate the tissue in a sculpted fashion. It should be noted that blackening or charring of the tissue is an undesirable result. This charred layer accumulates heat and transmits it to deeper tissue layers. A prolonged healing period could be required. By minimizing energy contact, impressions may be taken immediately. Preparation for the laminate veneers was initiated after the desired result was achieved (Fig.5).

A multistep preparation was used. The misaligned teeth (7, 9, and 11) were brought into proper arch form. Then appropriate guide cuts were made on teeth 4 through 13. Full preparation was finished (Fig. 6). At this time, an alginate impression was taken and poured in quick-set plaster. This plaster model allowed greater scrutiny as to the appropriateness of the preparations. Next, additional modifications were performed. The fiber from the Nd:YAG laser was placed under the gingiva for gingival sulcular troughing to provide an accurate representation of the cervical margin of the prepared teeth (Fig. 7). A full-arch impergum and permadyne impression was taken, as were a counter and a bite registration. All-Bond 2 (Bisco, Itasca, IL) was placed over the prepared teeth to minimize postoperative sensitivity. Diflunisal (1000 mg) was prescribed. The patient left the office feeling comfortable and without any bleeding or swelling. A postoperative tele-

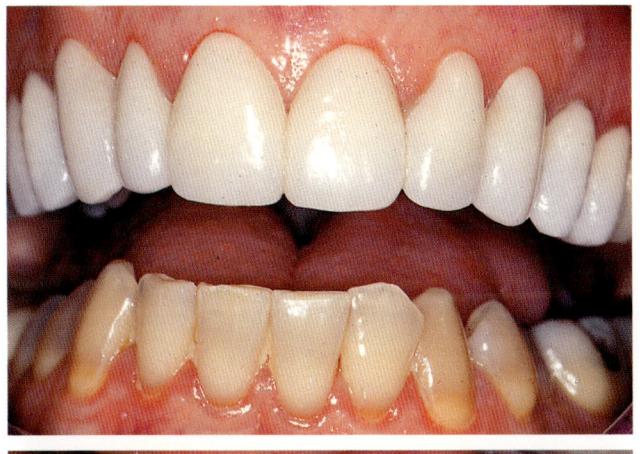

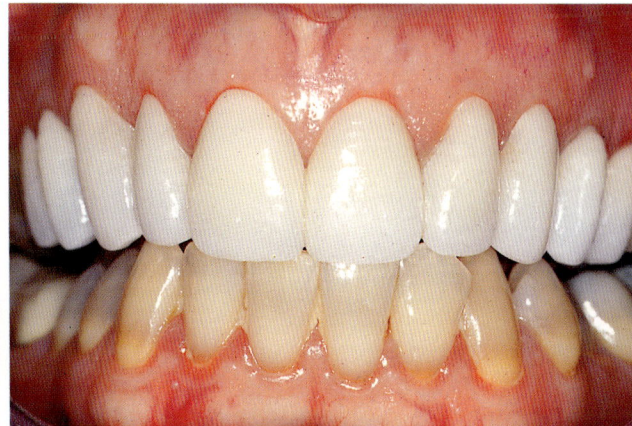

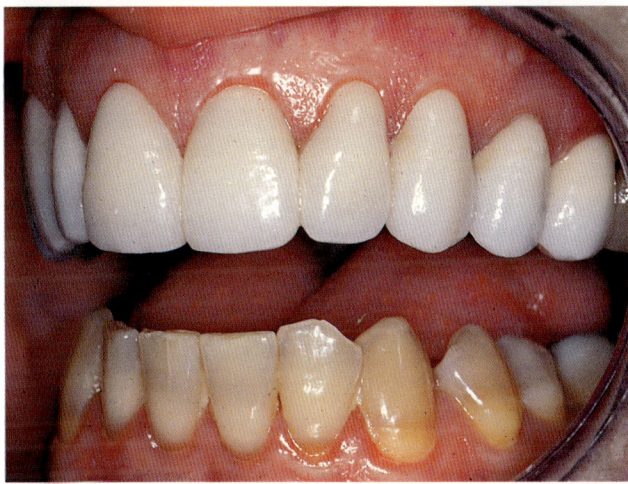

Fig. 11. Final postoperative result. Note the cosmetic gingival contour.

phone call 8 hours later confirmed her continued comfort.

Two days later, the patient returned to the operatory, and an infiltration of 72 mg of 2% lidocaine 1:50,000 epinephrine was administered to teeth 4 through 13. The postoperative gingival condition was satisfactory, and the desired gingival contour remained constant (Fig. 8). The porcelain laminates were tried in with Kerr Kolor Plus Plus A1 opaquer (Kerr Manufacturing, Romulus, MI) (Fig. 9). After try-in, the case was placed and cured with the HGM 100 argon bonding laser (HGM Medical Laser Systems, Salt Lake City, UT) (Fig. 10). Each argon pulse was delivered at 0.5 W for 10 seconds. After rapid curing, excess composite was removed, and occlusal equilibration for teeth 4 through 13 was established. The patient was satisfied with the final results of both her laminate veneers and the aesthetic appearance of the gingiva (Figs. 11 and 12).

Discussion

The use of a laser for gingivoplasty and gingival sulcular troughing instead of traditional scalpels, electrosurgery, or retraction cord is not new. It has been used for many years [3•,14••,16,17•,21••,22••,23,24]. The decision to use a laser in this case was based on several factors. The laser provided greater accuracy in sculpting the gingival margin. Throughout the procedure, the surgical site remained relatively free from bleeding and clearly visible. The inflammatory infiltrate was less with the laser than it would have been with electrosurgery [25]. Sterility of the surgical site was also better with the laser compared with a scalpel. Postoperative swelling was minimal. These factors also allowed impressions to be taken immediately for the laminate veneers.

For years, bonding laminate veneers onto teeth has been achieved with the curing lamp. Its disadvantages were not emphasized because there was no other technology with which to compare it. For multiple veneer placement, the curing lamp needs more exposure time. In our case study, the curing lamp might have needed 12 to 20 minutes of exposure time. This would have produced great heat with possible overload and temporary shut down of the unit. The patient may also have experienced this heat on her skin or mucous membranes. Occasional movement of the veneers could have occurred during this long exposure time. The decision to use the argon bonding laser

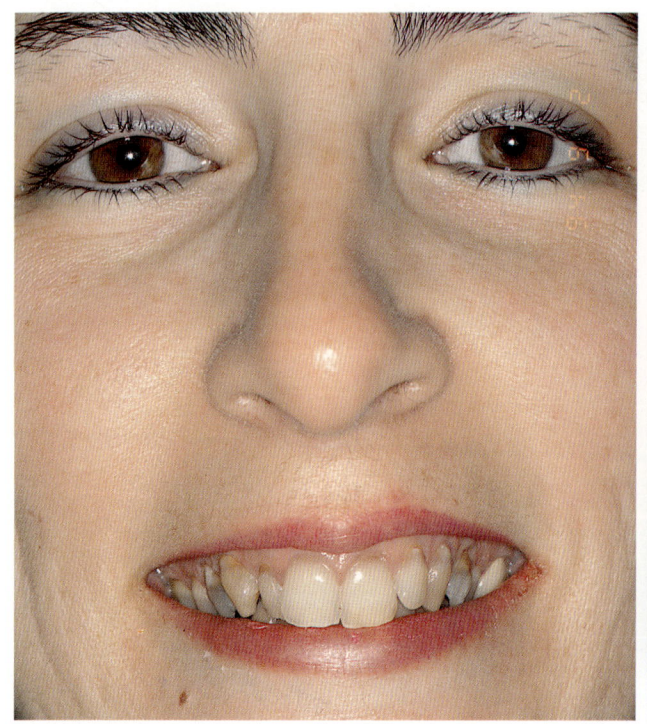

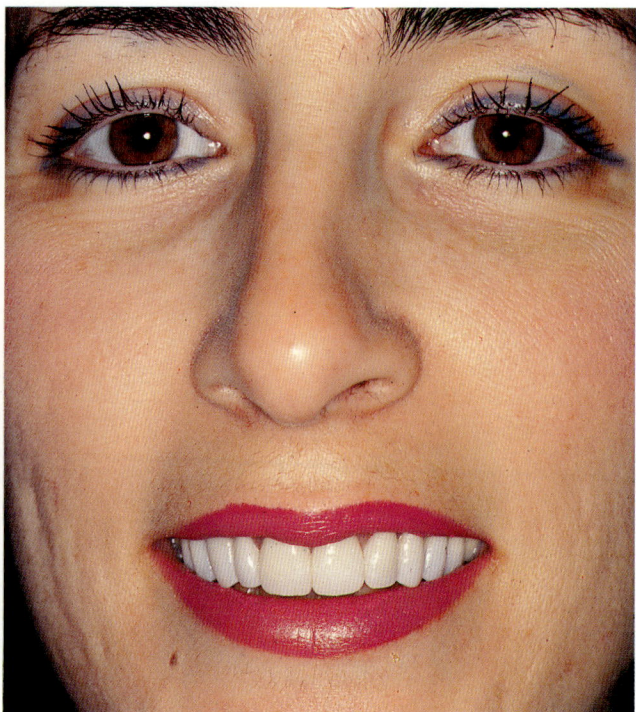

Fig. 12. Preoperative (*left panel*) and postoperative (*right panel*) full-face views.

was based on several factors. We wanted a faster cure of the composite. Average curing of composites occurs within 10 seconds. The argon laser also achieves a deeper and more even cure than the conventional bonding lamp [26••]. There is no heat for the patient to perceive.

Conclusions

case study demonstrates the effectiveness of dental lasers in conventional cosmetic dental treatment. Of the five commercially available dental lasers, we have discussed two wavelengths. These lasers have the ability to sculpt tissue, arrest bleeding, create a sterile surgical field, maintain constant clear visibility of the surgical site, keep postoperative pain and swelling to a minimum, and cure composite resins rapidly and deeply. Much research is being done to broaden the applications of lasers in dentistry [27•]. Their use on bone and tooth structure has already been shown to be effective, although it has not yet been approved by the US Food and Drug Administration.

Acknowledgments

I gratefully acknowledge the following companies, which provided support for this article: McAndrews/Restoradent/Somar Dental Laboratories for assistance with the porcelain laminate veneers; Kerr Dental Manufacturing for providing Porcelite; Excel Technology for providing their Nd:YAG dental laser system; HGM for providing their portable composite-curing argon dental laser unit. I also want to thank Nancy Marcelli for the long, hard hours she put in as a dental assistant.

References and recommended reading

Papers of particular interest, published within the annual period of review, have been highlighted as:
- •   Of special interest
- •• Of outstanding interest

1. Cobb CM, McCawley TK, Killoy WJ: **A preliminary study on the effect of the Nd:YAG laser on the root surfaces and subgingival microflora in vivo.** *J Periodontol* 1992, 63:701–707.

2. Pick RM: **Using lasers in clinical dental practice.** *J Am Dent Assoc* 1993, 124:37–47.
•
This paper gives a general overview of the uses of lasers in dentistry. It is helpful as a foundation for the clinician who is unfamiliar with the benefits lasers can offer.

3. White JM, Goodie HE, Rose CL: **Use of the pulsed Nd:YAG laser for intraoral soft tissue surgery.** *Lasers Surg Med* 1991, 11:455–461.
•
The application of an Nd:YAG laser is compared with that of a conventional scalpel in dental soft-tissue surgery. Surgical procedures are evaluated with respect to periodontal pocket depths, degree of pain, bleeding, inflammation, and need for anesthesia.

4. Smith TA, Thompson JA, Lee WE: **Patient response to dental laser treatment: a preliminary report.** *J Calif Dent Assoc* 1991, 19:37–38, 40–41.
•
This article studies patient responses to and acceptance of the laser. A survey of 263 patients treated with lasers addressed anxiety, fear, discomfort, and pain.

5. Myers TM: **Laser light in the oral cavity.** *Natural Science: At Edge.* April 1992:236–239.
••
This article presents an overview of lasers in general. It covers the different types of lasers and their application. It is a good paper for the clinician who wishes to get a broad, basic concept about lasers.

6. Ny, Springer, Vertage: **Nd:YAG laser therapy in dental and oral surgery.** In *Advances in Nd:YAG Laser Surgery.* Tokyo: Atinora Nagasawa MD Department of Oral Surgery, Metropolitan Hiroo General Hospital; 1988:235–246.

7. Maiman TH: **Stimulated optical radiation in ruby.** *Nature* 1960, **187**:493–494.

8. Stern RH, Renger HL, Howell FV: **Laser effects on vital dental pulps.** *Br Dent J* 1969, **127**:26–28.

9. Adrian JC, Bernier JL, Sprague WG: **Laser and the dental pulp.** *J Am Dent Assoc* 1971, **83**:113–117.

10. Adrian JC: **Pulp effects of neodymium laser: a preliminary report.** *Oral Surg Oral Med Oral Pathol* 1977, **44**:301–305.

11. Pick RM, Pecaro BC, Silberman CJ: **The laser gingivectomy: the use of the CO_2 laser for the removal of phenytoin hyperplasia.** *J Periodontol* 1985, **56**:492–496.

12. Tuffin JR, Carruth JAS: **The carbon dioxide surgical laser.** *Br Dent J* 1980, **149**:255–258.

13. **Dental applications of advanced lasers.** Burlington: JGM Associates; 1992.
••
This book gives the clinician a detailed history involving the physics, applications, types, and advantages of dental lasers, as well as recent advances in the field. It is well-organized and can be used easily as a reference.

14. Roed P: **The potential use of CO_2 laser gingivectomy for phenytoin induced gingival hyperplasia in mentally retarded patients.** *J Clin Periodontol* 1993, **20**:729–731.
••
This paper studies the use of the CO_2 in gingivectomy for phenytoin-induced gingival hyperplasia in mentally retarded patients. Despite it narrow focus, however, it affords the clinician an overall understanding of the advantages of laser use.

15. Nemeth JR: **Use both Nd:YAG and CO_2 lasers.** *Dent Econ* 1992, **82**:79–83.

16. Myers TD, Myers WD, Stone RM: **First soft tissue study utilizing a pulsed Nd:YAG dental laser.** *Northwest Dent* 1989, **68**:14–17.

17. Epstein S: **Curettage revisited: laser therapy.** *Pract Periodontics Aesthet Dent* 1992, **4**:27–31.
•
Describes the use of the Nd:YAG laser for gingival curettage. The technique described is uncomplicated and may result in less patient discomfort than conventional curettage. Four case summaries are presented.

18. Stein E, Sedlacek T, Fabian RL, Nishioka NS: **Acute and chronic effects of bone ablation with a pulsed holmium laser.** *Lasers Surg Med* 1990, **10**:384–388.

19. Powell L, Kelsey P, Blankenau R, Barkmeier W: **The use of an argon laser for polymerization of composite resin.** *J Esthet Dent* 1989, **1**:34–37.

20. Powell GL, Morton TH, Whisenant BK: **Argon laser oral safety parameters for teeth.** *Lasers Surg Med* 1993, **13**:548–552.

21. Miller PD Jr: **Periodontal plastic surgery.** *Curr Opin Periodontol* 1993, **1**:136–143.
••
Describes many soft-tissue surgical techniques. The clinician will find this article helpful in evaluating patients for surgery.

22. Pick RM, Colvard MD: **Current status of lasers in soft tissue dental surgery.** *J Periodontol* 1993, **64**:589–602.
••
This paper brings the clinician up to date on soft-tissue applications of lasers. A good article for the clinician wishing to incorporate lasers into his or her dental practice.

23. Myers TD, Murphy DG, White JM, Gold SI: **Conservative soft tissue management with the low-powered pulsed Nd:YAG dental laser.** *Pract Periodontics Aesthet Dent* 1992, **4**:6–12.

24. Gold SI, Vilardi MA: **Effect of Nd:YAG laser curettage on gingival crevicular tissues.** *J Dent Res* 1992, **71**:299.

25. Pick RM: **Comparative wound healing of the scalpel, Nd:YAG laser and electrosurgery in oral mucosa.** In *Innovation et technologie en biologie et medicine: actes du deuxieme congres mondial. L'impact des lasers en sciences odontologiques.* Paris: 1990:105.

26. Hinoura K, Miyazaki M, Onose H: **Influence of argon laser curing on resin bond strength.** *Am J Dent* 1993, **6**:69–71.
••
The argon laser is now being used to cure composites, with very good results. This article elaborates on this topic in an articulate manner.

27. Powell GL: **Lasers in the limelight: what will the future bring?** *J Am Dent Assoc* 1992, **123**:71–74.
•
This article addresses what might happen in the near future in the field of dental lasers. It discusses some important ideas, including hard- and soft-tissue applications of the laser.

Dr. Harvey Passes, 1360 Northern Boulevard, Suite 107, Manhasset, NY 11030, USA.

Marketing the cosmetic practice via television

Richard N. Smith, DMD, and Mary E. Naslund Smith, BS

Springfield, Oregon, USA

Everyone is marketing their dental practice whether they know it or not. It is far better to design the desired effect than to send mixed messages to your clients. All marketing must be carried out with a plan or mission that is internalized by the doctor and by each member of the staff. The mission coupled with creative talent becomes the proprietary personality of your office and the focus of your marketing efforts. Internal marketing is perhaps the most economical and effective—and most used—method of creating positive results for the practice. External marketing takes your office out to the public most often in print via newsletters, direct mailings, and the yellow pages. Getting the message out through newspapers, radio, and television has and will become increasingly important. This article takes you through the steps we used to identify and market to our cosmetic clients. The results of our demographic and psychographic studies afford unique insight into the type of person attracted by our services. Marketing to this group has to do with diversity in appeal, "the boomers," and experiential motivation.

For some of us, marketing is the "M" word. It is not to be mentioned in polite company and certainly not among your dental peers. There is a long-held bias in the dental community against promoting one's own dental practice. Fear of censure by the local dental society and the threat of possible legal or ethical disputes keep many from promoting their unique office [1]. It is true, however, that you are marketing now whether you intend to or not. The question in effect is whether you planned it or it planned you.

Whether you call it internal or external, aggressive or passive, team building or staff training, education or bringing up alternatives, it is marketing. The only difference is in the desired results. If you have a plan or system that you act on consistently and honestly, every day and every year, you will obtain the result you desire. Just be certain you understand what results your actions are having in the community and the market place.

In March 1994, the Journal of the American Dental Association published an interesting article about professional and patient views of dentistry [2•]. The authors found that patients' beliefs about their own dentist are more positive than the dentists' own views of themselves, and that dentists believe they are not equal to their own view of the ideal dentist. The good news is that the vast majority of patients like their present dentist. The bad news is that we as dentists don't believe it. This germ of self doubt is like a virus implanted into the psyche of all dentists. Only a few of us ever recover. We encourage the cosmetic dentistry profession to seek recovery and start to act like the respected professionals we are. We have become our own worst enemy, and this has blocked our need to educate our patients about their unique dental possibilities. This need should be met with a thoughtful yet persistent attitude and with our own egos intact.

Internal marketing is one of our most powerful means of improving our office productivity and financial health. Austin [3] has written much about marketing the cosmetic practice, and her advice has centered on the immediate impact that you have on your patients. First impressions are lasting. If you are holding yourself and your office out to the public as *the* cosmetic dental center for your area, then your staff and "systems" have to be exceptional and in place. Don't talk the talk if you can't walk the walk.

The vision

Tools and information are not proprietary. They are open to anyone who wants to use them. The systems (software) and the equipment (hardware) are available to anyone who bellies up to the bar, pays the price, and puts them to use. The truly exceptional practice is the one that has taken the time create a "vision" or "mission." That mission must fit into the personal lives of all the team members, doctor and staff. What is proprietary about your office is your "office personality,"

Abbreviation
ADI—area of dominant influence.

or "integrated mission." That personality is the motor behind the application and utilization of the systems and equipment you have in place (King, Lecture presented at American Academy of Cosmetic Dentistry Annual Meeting, Phoenix, 1994).

There is an anonymous poem that tells the fable of the lion and the rabbit:

A lion met a tiger

As they drank beside a pool.

Said the tiger, "Tell me why

You're roaring like a fool."

"That's not foolish," said the lion

With a twinkle in his eyes.

"They call me king of all the beasts

Because I advertise!"

A rabbit heard them talking

And ran home like a streak.

He thought he'd try the lion's plan,

But his roar was just a squeak.

A fox came to investigate,

Had luncheon in the woods.

Moral: When you advertise, my friends,

Be sure you've got the goods!

You can have all the finest systems and equipment, but unless you have the personal skills, you will be doomed to repeat the same failure patterns. Get training and personal counseling. There exist many excellent advisors and counselors in every area of the world, and we are sure there is one not far from you.

Your first and most important task in developing a marketing system is to put together jointly with your staff and advisor a mission for the office and implement it seamlessly (Reed, Lecture presented at Excellence in Dentistry Seminar, Sun River, 1994). Then and only then will you build a practice that gives no mixed messages and truly treats your clients as you yourself would want to be treated.

Define your market

In this article, however, we would like to offer an understanding of *external marketing* of a cosmetic practice, which takes the concept to new heights. The traditional approach of relying almost exclusively on limited direct mail or yellow page advertising can be expanded to include other print media, radio, and television. In reviewing the literature, we find very little that deals completely with external advertising beyond traditional and narrow views. We follow the literature with a certain bent. Not much has been done in dentistry, much less cosmetic dentistry, with regard to mature adult marketing, or especially "experiential" or "psychographic" targeting. The mature market is blooming, not just booming, and it is most susceptible to this kind of advertising. As a consequence, everyone who wants to delve into this form of marketing has to reinvent the wheel time and time again. Therefore, we present our individual experience at combining the most effective media—newspaper, radio, and television—in a coordinated effort to reach the largest mature audience possible.

The first thing we did was conduct a survey of our top patients. Reed (Excellence in Dentistry Seminar, 1994) and King (American Academy of Cosmetic Dentistry Annual Meeting, 1994) both espoused this method as an excellent way to get to know your practice and its most valuable assets, *ie*, your top 100 patients. Both said that if you and your staff sit together and patiently select, by popular opinion, your most enjoyable clients and limit the number to your favorite 100, you will have the key to your practice's success. These people will be not only your biggest source of referrals but also your largest source of income for the practice. By identifying these top 100 patients and all the others they have referred to your practice in the past year, you will have found 80% of your annual income. That means that the other 20% of your income came from the rest of the practice population.

Covey [4] set forth an excellent way of bringing this point home. He recommended that you divide your business life into four equal squares and label each one individually as 1) urgent and important, 2) not urgent but important, 3) urgent but not important, and 4) not urgent and not important. He asserted that we spend only 20% on square two. Our most productive and meaningful time is spent in square two, however, and it routinely delivers 80% of our meaningful income. The point is that if we can just spend more time in square two (not urgent but important), our lives will be greatly enriched financially and spiritually. If we could just spend more time with our top 100 patients and their referrals, then our lives would be far less stressful and more greatly rewarding.

Gathering data

The results of our demographic survey surprised us. We thought the majority of our patients had been local, *ie*, that they came to us because of our location in their neighborhood. Notable was the distance traveled by most of the top patients. The majority traveled relatively great distances from different neighborhoods and towns to come to our office (Table 1). Also notable to us was the fact that more than half of our top 100 clients were referred by word of mouth. The next most common source was from our previously limited print advertising (Fig. 1). Way down the list, and insignificant, was our yellow page ad.

Table 1. Age of cosmetic dentistry patients, and distance traveled to dentist's office*

Median age: 49 years
Average age: 47.5 years
Distance traveled
   10+ miles: 16 patients
   3–5 miles: 7 patients
   0–2 miles: 5 patients

*Based on a survey of 100 patients (Smith, Unpublished data).

Income levels were fairly evenly distributed from less than $10,000 to more than $70,000 a year, but the majority made in excess of $40,000. Life styles were also fairly similar. The top five favorite activities of all respondents were travel; walking, camping, and hiking; music; fitness; and the arts. We live in the beautiful state of Oregon, where hunters and fishermen are a dime a dozen, but hunting and fishing were down the list. The most significant finding of the survey was the median age of the top patients: approximately 49 years (Table 1).

The boomers are coming

Why is age such a *significant marker* for today's cosmetic practice? The boomers are coming! Of primary importance to all in the practice of dentistry today is the need to understand the psychographics of the mature population. (For those to whom *psychographics* is a new word, please read on. We hope to make this clearer as we progress through this article).

We hired a consultant, Mr. John Rude of Age Matters, Inc. [5], to spend a day at our office and help the entire team get acquainted with their own built-in prejudices and feelings about older people and aging in general. We jointly discovered that humanity has spent the past

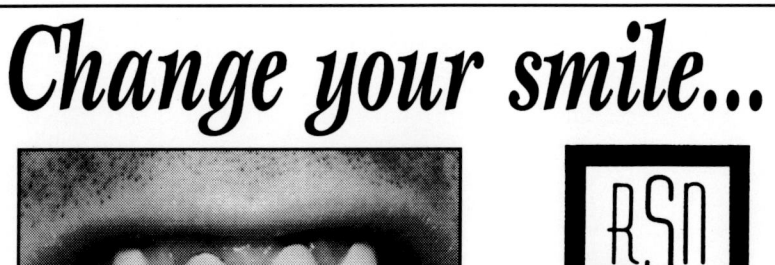

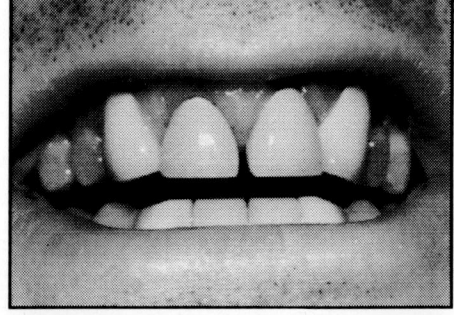

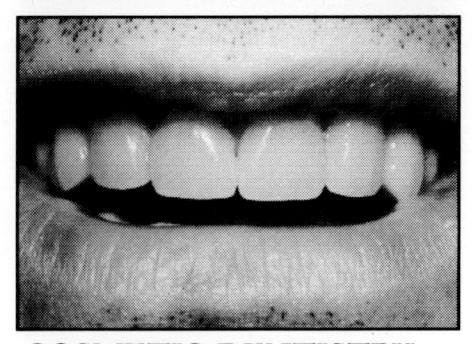

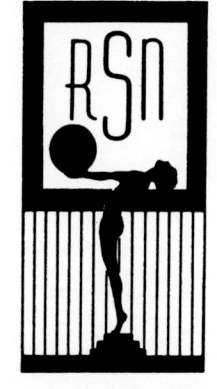

Fig. 1. Example of an old print advertisement used prior the video-radio-print combination.

2000 years trying to make people live longer and better lives. We did it, but now we are embarrassed by them. We asked the members of a focus group the following question: "What were the major obstacles, issues or barriers you needed to overcome before you made up your mind to go forward (with cosmetic dental care)?" One member of the group replied, "I was told by my previous dentist, 'What do you expect for a person your age?' "

Some important statistics need to be brought up here (Table 2). The overall rise in the population density of mature adults combined with the fact that the vast majority of them have most of their teeth still in function is significant. The need for replacement of defective and worn out restorations (mostly amalgam) and for progressive periodontal therapy is going to be overwhelming in this population. Wake up, people! There is no shortage of work to be done. It has ever been thus: if it's broken, fix it, and if it bleeds, stop it. Function used to lead, but now it's cosmetics (Christensen, Lecture presented at the American Academy of Cosmetic Dentistry Annual Meeting, Miami, 1993).

Table 2. The aging of the American population and the future of the cosmetic dentistry market

In the 1990s:
  The population of consumers aged 18–34 years will decline by 7.8 million
  The population of consumers aged 40–74 years will grow by 19.9 million, of whom more than 18 million will be 40–59 years old
By the year 2000:
  13% of the population will be older than 65 years
  12% of the population will be older than 75 years
In the next 30 years:
  The population aged 50 years or older will increase 74%
  The population aged 50 years or younger will increase 1%
Functional teeth of the population aged 65–75 years

Decade	1960s	1980s	1990s	2000s
Teeth, n	7.4	17.9	20	20+

Understanding the mature market

We, as a profession, need to understand this growing demographic group because it brings into focus an entirely new method of looking at a group of diverse people. The traditional marketing and advertising method was to target a potential consumer by age or other easy means of segregation, eg, religion, income, education, neighborhood, or routine habits. Now it is becoming more important to rely on experimental or psychographic segmentation based on behavior, or better yet, motivation.

Everyone is motivated in some way. What motivates one person may not motivate another, but we are all motivated by something. Your office team has vastly different motivational resources, just as yours varies from theirs. The world is eclectic. So is the mature adult market.

What motivates the 18- to 25-year-old age group does not motivate 55- to 70-year-olds (if you can even call them a group). There are certain experiences that may be shared within all groups, but it is more likely that these experiences occur at certain age levels more than at others. The younger you are, the more likely you are to be involved with image or identity, eg, cars or clothes. The more mature you are, the more likely you are to be involved with social issues and connectedness, eg, spirituality or ecological issues.

Ageism

We need to examine our own view of the aging process. The commonly held view is the "deficit view." This can be, and is often, a self-fulfilling prophecy. We see life as a progression or advancement up to a certain age, after which it is all downhill. The certain age, after which it is all downhill. The common phrase "over the hill" is a classic "ageist" attitude. We have all reveled in the typical black-balloon, coffin-adorned 40th birthday celebration. We are not against humor, but we need to examine how deep-seated this idea really is and how much of an effect it has on our own sense of where we are in life. To some the glass is half empty. This is the deficit view: you have finished half already and have little left to drink. To the new mind it is half full; you have filled it only half way and have to go and get more.

The upcoming attitude toward aging is found in the "life span development view." In this paradigm, aging is a lifelong process, with gains and losses throughout. There continues to be an opportunity to learn from loss, alter behaviors, and develop capacities. Instead of a steady rise followed by inexorable decline, this view sees life as a series of continually rising steps, each one taking you to greater heights.

In expanding the office's attitude about aging, our consultant helped to conduct a "focus group" selected from our top 100 patients. A focus group is essentially a method of gathering qualitative consumer information. The format encourages confidentiality and trust, fun and work, and ease of sharing and dialogue as each participant draws from the energy, comments, and ideas of the others. Obviously, we could not have all 100 participate in the focus group; we therefore limited it to around 10. All of these patients had experienced cosmetic dentistry at the office and could talk about the experience from their particular points of view. Their median age was 50 years, and they came from a cross section of skills and professions.

Ten discussion questions were presented. (Answers to and the resultant message from the first question are available in Table 3). Rude summarized some of the messages from the focus group in this way:

Outcomes clearly demonstrated that the work being accomplished is in the realm of transforming people's lives; especially the way they perceive themselves.—A real challenge to advertising will be to effectively communicate this service in a manner that captures the power of altering people's lives (transformation) as opposed to the obvious (physiology & function).

The key for advertising will be to capture the psychology of the customer's experience.

Finally, cosmetic dentistry needs a new language, a new definition, simply because the word cosmetic doesn't convey the power of this work.

The argument could be presented that if I am going to market to the top 100, why advertise externally? Why complicate my life? Why? Why not? There might be a better top 100!

Quality and psychographics

Kennedy [6•] (Paper presented at the Excellence in Dentistry Seminar, Sun River, 1994) stated that for demand to exceed supply, you must have reliable, predictable, consistent systems that affordably and efficiently provide abundant quantities of quality prospects, customers, and clients.

Quality is the key word here. If you can devise a system that consistently provides quality patients then you ought to look at it. Developing coordinated print, radio, and television advertising constitutes the most powerful way to find abundant quantities of quality clients.

One of the great results of involvement with the mature market is that any advertisement developed from an experiential view is ageless; *ie*, it is not demographic, but rather, psychographic (*ie*, behavioral, motivational, additudinal) [7]. People of all ages can relate to the experience of desiring improved dental health and appearance. The message or advertisement is a learning experience for the viewer, listener, or reader.

Public relations versus advertising

Our experience with an advertising agency began with a discussion of the difference between public relations and advertising. These are different forms of marketing and deliver different results under different time tables. Public relations makes the client base larger because more are aware of the services you and your fellow professionals can provide. Advertising makes your own client base larger. A simple analogy is that public relations makes the pie bigger so all can enjoy a bigger piece, whereas advertising makes your piece of the pie bigger regardless of the numbers of others sharing the pie. Public relations takes a commitment in time, whereas advertising brings results quickly and directly to you. Our personal opinion is that life is short; we wanted the biggest bang for our dollar *now*.

We have to relate an experience that one of our dentist friends had with an attempt at public relations. He was on a local radio talk show, something like "Ask an Expert." When introducing him, the radio host referred to him as a specialist in cosmetic dentistry. A disgruntled dentist from out of town reported the incident, and our friend ended up being censured by his local and state dental organizations. Remember, no one is allowed to represent themselves as a specialist unless that specialty is recognized by the American Dental Association.

The moral here is that despite your altruistic attempts to increase the size of the pie for all, you could be inadvertently chastised for your behavior. Omer Reed (Lecture presented at Excellence in Dentistry Seminar, 1994) once said that if dentists were told to form a firing squad, they would do it in a circle.

Mixed messages

Important in any discussion of print, radio, and television advertising is the quality of final product. One cannot deliver a mixed message and come out unscathed. For example, if you openly promote your asepsis as the best that dentistry can offer, but your windows are dirty and there are stains on the reception area carpet, your message is lost.

Creative talent is a must. No matter how clever you think you may be, outside talent is essential in developing creative ideas to influence your experiential market. If you are representing your team and office as exceptional, then your advertisement should be exceptional. Don't spare the dollar on the quality of video presentation. An additional consideration, however, should be the ability to modify the message easily and affordably. If your voice and media talent can't go with the flow of your results, then you may be doomed to ever increasing costs of modification and alteration of the initial message. Know what you want. Communicate what your want. Be sure you and your agency agree on what you want before you buy it. Simple informal presentation of your video as conceived by your talent and agency is advisable before you commit your money.

Area of dominant influence

Before you have gone all the way to production, you must have previously discussed the cost of running the advertisement. The area of dominant influence (ADI) and frequency must be included in such a discussion. ADIs have different values. ADIs in New York or Los Angeles have greater value than in Springfield, Oregon, or Charlotte, North Carolina. The cost of the voiceover and video production team is also influenced by the ADI. ADI seems to be a self-explanatory term, but it needs to be interpreted for the novice. If you lived in our area of the world, ie, Springfield, Oregon, the cost of advertising would be modified by the size of the potential audience reached. The number of potential viewers watching your TV advertisement influences the cost of advertising. The reach and influence of your local television channels have an effect on the overall cost of running your advertisement. The more you will potentially influence, the higher the cost of running your advertisement. This cost can be modified by limiting your reach to local cable stations and smaller community publications, a wise way to test your advertisement in the community. If it isn't doing what you want, then inexpensively modify it. It all needs to be built in at the beginning.

Frequency

Frequency is all important. We are sure that many of us have attempted to get the message out about our unique practice but quit before the message was heard and thus determined that the media weren't for us. The adage states that for every three times an advertisement is run, only one gets through to the mind of the intended recipient [8]. A message requires at least nine exposures to sink in. If you want to get to your intended audience, give them the courtesy of exposure to your message at least 27 times. This is true of direct mail, newspaper, or television.

In your dealing with media gurus, play by these rules, and you will get your intended result. You must know the total cost of production and runs before you begin this course of marketing. You should also address and learn the definitive range of the cost of modifying the advertisement.

Results

Our own advertisements produced astounding results. They were run with proper frequency and on appropriately directed television channels and sections of the newspaper. A 2-week run on television and in the newspaper resulted in an increase of quality clients far exceeding our power to see them. In 2 weeks, we had received our normal month's flow of new patients. An increase in new patients means nothing unless it turns into meaningful delivery of new services. Our average weekly production increased by more than 25% during the following 3 months. We ran this campaign twice in 2 months in the spring of 1994, and we were still resting on the spin off of this system during the autumn.

This system works. It is a no-brainer, and we shall run it again in the near future. It meets the criteria of Kennedy's [6•] admonition that it be reliable, predictable, and consistent, and that it provide abundant quantities of quality patients.

Table 3. Attitudes of cosmetic dentistry patients toward their treatment*

Sample question
What were the major barriers to overcome before you accepted treatment?
    Trust in the profession
    Self-esteem
    Past experiences
    Vanity
    Financial considerations

Consultant's summary of patients' responses
In our consumer-driven society, it is easy to compromise self for things or other people. People will put up with deformities and actually alter who they are (*ie*, their inner selves) and the way they are being (*ie*, their outer selves) to accommodate their personal image. People come into the office with all kinds of conditions and preconceived notions that involve distrust, low self esteem, and resentments. Personal needs often get put on the back burner.

*Based on discussions with 10 patients (Smith, Unpublished data).

Conclusions

We need to make one thing absolutely clear. No one can create a need where none existed before. The ability to do so would constitute a form of abuse. For some inexplicable reason, some of us in this world still believe it is possible. It may be for this reason alone that some of us view marketing or advertising as the unethical or evil control of others' minds. Although television and the print media are powerful, they cannot create need!

Farran [9••], founder of Dental Mania, was right when he said, "A Grand Canyon of ignorance exists between us over here on the supply side and the American people across the chasm on the demand side." The need is there already. The information is just not available. The question is, do we want to direct the needy toward us, or do we want to inform them about the possibilities? The answer is both. Excellent public relations combined with excellent advertising is the ideal solution for marketing cosmetic services. Public relations directed at informing the populace about the nature and process of cosmetic dental services combined with a direct call to seek the service at your office is best.

We are currently involved with the American Academy of Cosmetic Dentistry, along with a few of its accredited members in the process of developing such a public relations campaign. As Rude and Adams [5] found, "Cosmetic dentistry needs a new language, a new definition, simply because the word *cosmetic* doesn't convey the power of this work."

Dentists as a group need to become more assertive in the marketplace. There exists a blur out there in the media. We are all subject to it, and we need to stand out. We have patients who like us and who have a need that cries out to be filled. Those of us who do promote the profession by providing information about possibilities, either internally or externally, need to be commended for increasing the size of the pie we all eat. Remember: knowledge is not proprietary; personality is [3]. We all need to share the knowledge.

Cooperative collaboration between a large professional organization and individual providers of proven skills could produce a large synergistic effect. Not only would the pie get bigger, but for those so inclined to promote their practice, the piece could be exponentially bigger, and your top 100 could truly be tops!

Why not?

References and recommended reading

Papers of particular interest, published within the annual period of review, have been highlighted as:
- Of special interest
- •• Of outstanding interest

1. Smith CJ: **Don't blow your own horn.** *N Y State Dent J* 1993, **59**:72–73.

2. • Gerbert B, Bleecker T, Saub E: **Dentists and the patients who love them.** *J Am Dent Assoc* 1994, **125**:264–272.
An excellent article about our patient base and what patients think about their dentist. Provides insight on how our patients rate professional qualities and how we rate ourselves against our ideal. Median age is again approaching 50 among responding dentists and patients.

3. Austin C: *Cosmetic Dentistry: Systems and Strategies, a Step by Step Guide for Incorporating Cosmetic Dentistry Into the General Dentistry Practice*, edn 2. Minneapolis: C Austin; 1992.

4. Covey S: *The Seven Habits of Highly Effective People.* New York: Simon and Schuster, 1989.

5. Rude J, Adams C: **Marketing to older Americans** *The Business News*, August-September 1993:35–36.

6. • Kennedy D: *How To Solve All Your Advertising, Marketing, and Sales Problems Fast and Forever.* Phoenix: Empire Communications Corp.; 1994.
Dan Kennedy is a nationally known speaker on marketing and he promotes his own books and tapes on marketing. This is a no-holds-barred, no-nonsense, straightforward look at all the strategies needed to enact and run an effective marketing system.

7. Wolfe D: *Serving the Ageless Market.* New York: McGraw-Hill; 1990.

8. Levinson JC: *Guerrilla Marketing Attack.* Boston: Houghton Mifflin Co.; 1989.

9. •• Farran H: **More beautiful than you were born.** *Am Acad Cosmetic Dent J* Spring 1994:34–36.
Farran really hits the nail on the head with this article on external marketing for the dental profession. He points out that we need to discuss forthrightly with our patients their dental options and possibilities and make a wave in the blur of advertising that all of us sit through. We are liked and respected, according to the author, and patients will listen if we just take the time to give them the information they so desperately need.

Richard N. Smith, DMD, 5811 Main Street, Suite D, Springfield, OR 97478, USA.

Differing porcelain systems

David M. Schneider, DMD, MScD

Swampscott, Massachusetts, USA

Current research in ceramics has centered on improving the strength, fit, and bondability of porcelain. Several different approaches to accomplishing these ends have led to the development of stronger cores, castable glass, computer-generated restorations, and chemically altered basic ceramics. Improvements in these basic parameters of clinical success have led to the use of all-ceramic systems such as inlays, onlays, conservative veneers, anterior and posterior crowns, and even fixed partial dentures. Porcelain veneers and full-coverage ceramic crowns have held up well clinically. Porcelain inlays and fixed partial dentures have presented problems with fit and strength, respectively, that may need correcting before they are clinically predictable in all situations. Nevertheless, it is apparent that modern dental porcelain technology has come a long way since it was originally introduced as an esthetic replacement for less cosmetic, metal-based restorations.

Porcelain is a material of contrasts. The light shining through an unbonded porcelain veneer shows us its potential fragility. Observing glassy-smooth mandibular teeth worn down by a porcelain maxillary reconstruction reminds us of its hardness. Porcelain has been used for esthetics so long that its safety is virtually unquestioned [1], with the rare exception [2], and its versatility is such that it can be used anywhere in the mouth as a restorative material. The long-range clinical success of porcelain restorations depends on several factors, such as fracture toughness, fit, luting integrity, wear, surface smoothness, and esthetic matching. In an effort to address these issues clinically, several different systems have been developed over the years to improve the properties and performance of dental porcelain.

General research

Attempts to strengthen dental porcelains have taken several forms, from altering the basic chemistry of the porcelain to experimenting with techniques of its manipulation. Baker and Clark [3] tested a new, stronger type of glass matrix to surround the crystalline phase of the porcelain. In an attempt to develop a stronger ceramic implant, Kon and Kuwayuma [4] found that adding 10 wt % fine diamond particles increased the fracture toughness by three times over that of unaltered hydroxyapatite porcelain. Working with Ceramco II porcelain (Ceramco, Burlington, NJ), Denry et al. [5] used several surface coating ion exchange treatments and reported a significant increase in flexural strength. In a separate study of Dicor ceramics (Caulk Co., Milford, DE), Denry and Rosenstiel [6] incorporated lithium fluoride into the Dicor powder and increased flexural strength significantly at optimal temperatures. Evaluating the effect of tempering porcelain, Hojjatie and Anusavice [7], found that cooling porcelain in air or silicone oil from an initial temperature of 650° to 850°C improved the resistance to cracks and failure [7]. Akkas [8] found that conventional air cooling was best for glassy porcelains (Vita; Vita Zahnfabrik, Bad Saeckingen, FRG), and slow cooling in the furnace was best for crystalline porcelains (Ceramco).

Whereas basic studies in evaluating and improving the strength of porcelain continue, of perhaps more direct clinical relevance is the study by Mante et al. [9] on the lowering of fracture toughness of Vitadur N porcelain (Vident, Baldwin Park, CA) when tested in deionized water and artificial saliva versus air. They suggested further testing of newer porcelains using more clinically relevant techniques. Two other studies of great clinical significance found the flexural strength of porcelains is not diminished by the acid etching process that is so vital to our modern techniques [10,11•], and Hahn and Löst [12] described an ultrasonic method of shaping porcelain that produced a smoother surface,

---

Abbreviations
CAD—computer-aided design; **CAM**—computer-aided manufacture; **FPD**—fixed partial denture; **PFM**—porcelain-fused-to-metal.

fewer microcracks, and greater bonding strength than a diamond wheel.

Bonding of composite resin to porcelain is clinically important in the luting of the restoration of tooth structure and in the repair of fractured porcelain. Russell and Meiers [13••] found that Dicor treated with ammonium bifluoride etchant and silane produced a significantly greater bond than the same cast glass material treated with Etch-Free Primer (Parkell, Farmingdale, NY) and C&B Metabond (Parkell). And Suliman et al. [14••], mixing various surface treatments and bonding agents, found the most effective surface treatment of Vita VMK 68 542 body porcelain (Vita Zahnfabrik) was a combination of diamond roughening and hydrofluoric acid treatment (all surfaces were treated with silane). It is clear that for the present, both micromechanical retention and chemical adhesion are important for ideal bonding.

Porcelain is very wear-resistant [15], but as we have all observed, it can be very abrasive to opposing materials. Because many of the present porcelain systems require adjustment after luting, the surface smoothness of the porcelain must be reestablished by polishing in the mouth. Hulterström and Bergman [16] found the Soflex system (3M Dental Products, St. Paul, MN) and the Shofu porcelain laminate polishing kit (Shofu Dental Corp., Menlo Park, CA) were the most effective polishing systems and that Vita Mark I (Vita Zahnfabrik), Empress (Ivoclar North America, Amherst, NY), and Dicor MGC (Caulk Co.) were the most polishable porcelains, whereas Scurria and Powers [17], using Dicor MGC and Ceramco II, found that a combination of finishing diamond points and diamond polishing gels produced the smoothest surfaces for both materials, and an even smoother surface for the feldspathic Ceramco II than autoglazing.

Arguably, the major advantage of porcelain is esthetic quality. Complicating the sometimes clinically elusive "perfect" match, however, Monsénégo et al. [18], studying the fluorescence of natural teeth and shade guides, found the six shade guides tested did not give fluorescent readings close to those of natural teeth in the whole range of shades, and that shade guides of the same origin did not necessarily match each other.

Inlays and onlays

Although there may not be one ideal porcelain inlay or onlay preparation, several factors seem to be important: the internal aspects of the preparation should be rounded, there should be enough thickness of material, although not more than 1.5 to 2 mm of unsupported porcelain, and there should be a shoulder or butt finish line with no bevels [19,20]. The restorations should be etched, silanated, and bonded in place with resin and adhesive procedures to prevent microleakage [21].

As with more extensive all-porcelain restorations, one major problem with the integrity of porcelain inlays is microcrack generation under stress. Peters et al. [22] showed that internal cracks (unseen and undetected clinically) can be generated as soon as 55% to 60% of the fracture load is reached and can be further aggravated by natural flaws in the porcelain or areas of less rigid support (eg, low-modulus base cements). Marginal integrity is also important for the clinical success of porcelain inlays, because wear of the resin luting agent occurs, even when chemically bonded, especially in areas of function [23]. The greater the marginal gap, the greater the wear of the cementing medium, with hybrid cements wearing more than microfills [24••]. Also important are wear of the material itself and its effect on opposing materials.

Several different ceramic systems have been studied in the past year in regard to the above modalities. The computer-aided design (CAD) and computer-aided manufacture (CAM) system [25•], Cerec (Siemens Dental Corp., Bensheim, FRG) being the most popular, utilizes an optical reading of the tooth preparation, computer design of the restoration, and a direct carving of the inlays from ceramic blocks, such as Vita feldspathic porcelain (Vita Zahnfabrik) or Dicor MGC, a glass ceramic of mica flakes surrounded by a glass matrix [26]. It was introduced as a direct system, but Nathanson et al. [27•] described an indirect technique using a simple die, which was perhaps more suited to clinical practice [27•]. In two studies of marginal fit, Cerec inlays showed a mean opening of 169 μm [24••] and, more important, a mean cervical marginal opening of 195.4±95.7 μm on a die (with a range of 59 to 391 μm) in comparison with 48.9±34.2 μm for a gold inlay (Fig.1 and Table 1) [28••]. Moreover, inlays cut from the Vitabloc Mark II porcelain (Vita Zahnfabrik) fit significantly better than those made from the Dicor MGC ceramic block [26]. Empress, a pressed glass ceramic system, was evaluated for wear and fit. It wore significantly less than regular porcelain and castable glass and wore the opposing enamel the least of these three materials [23]. Of particular interest, polished Empress wore less than glazed Empress. The mean marginal opening of an Empress inlay at three locations on a die varied from 65 to 122 μm with very large ranges (Fig. 1 and Table 1) [28••].

Of clinical interest, Dicor (Caulk Co.), a cast glass system, demonstrated a wear curve similar to enamel in one study [23] and showed significantly less microleakage with etching and resin bonding than with simple cementation with zinc phosphate or resin without adhesive techniques [21]. In a 2-year clinical study, 23 of 25 Dicor inlays were found clinically acceptable although cemented with glass ionomer cement [29]. Of preliminary significance in the quest for a better fitting porcelain inlay, a new refractory die material was described with a coefficient of expansion matching that of Vita VMK 68 porcelain. The resulting inlays showed

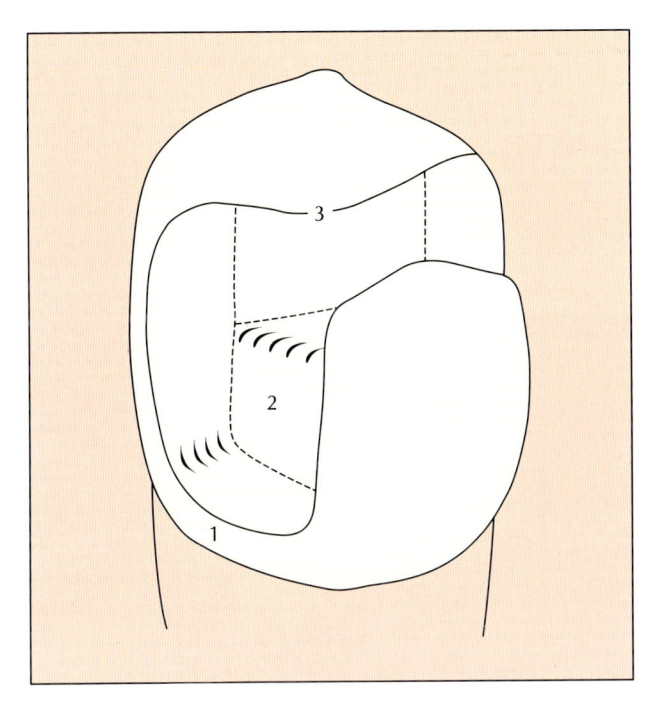

Fig. 1. Measuring locations for ceramic and gold inlays. 1—marginal area; 2—axial wall; 3—occlusal area. (*Modified from* Molin and Karlsson [28••].)

a mean marginal gap of 51.24 ± 20.84 µm against that of 100.43 ± 17.30 µm for the unmatched material [30].

Veneers

As porcelain veneers have become an important part of cosmetic treatment planning, it has been generally accepted that some preparation of the teeth is necessary for proper contours and fit. The fit of the veneer, as with any other restoration, is one of the keys to its clinical success. Sim and Ibbetson [31] studied the fit of veneers made from feldspathic porcelain (Vitadur N) using both a 0.021-mm platinum foil technique and a direct refractory die technique. In addition, two more sets of veneers were cast in Dicor, one of 0.5-mm, another of 1-mm thickness. They were measured at five locations (Fig. 2). In general, the fit of embedded, sectioned veneers showed the refractory die technique to have the best overall marginal fit. The authors believed that castable ceramics were not reliable enough for veneer fabrication. In another study of CAD-CAM (Cerec) veneers using Dicor MGC and Vita Mark II blocks compared with Vita VMK 68 porcelain fabricated on refractory dies, Liu *et al.* [32] found the greatest gap for all methods occurred in the incisal region and ranged from 103 to 117 µm. They concluded that after some internal surface grinding, the CAD-CAM veneers were as acceptable as those fabricated in the laboratory. An ancillary problem with the computer veneers, touched upon in the study, was the need to alter the color of the originally monochromatic ceramic blocks with shade modifiers under the veneers or surface stains over them.

A new porcelain veneer material (Colorlogic; Ceramco) with potentially improved masking characteristics has been described [33,34]. Barkmeier *et al.* [34] further tested the bonding of Colorlogic porcelain to enamel and dentin and found the bond to enamel was significantly higher than to dentin under any of six dentin bonding systems (39.0 ± 11.4 MPa for the enamel bond vs 27.2 ± 8.8 MPa for the best of the dentin bonding systems). Despite the improvements in dentin bonding, it

Table 1. Mean discrepancy between stone die–prepared tooth and inner surface of ceramic compared with gold inlays at three measuring points*

Measuring point	Inlay system	Stone die, µm Mean	SD	Range	Tooth, µm Mean	SD	Range
Marginal area	Gold	48.9	34.2	0–115	57.8	37.9	0–173
	Cerec†	195.4	95.7	59–391	155.3	106.9	32–369
	Mirage‡	84.7	64.4	0–279	128.0	108.7	0–407
	Empress§	65.4	59.0	0–256	114.7	105.2	0–469
Axial wall	Gold	63.8	32.9	18–173	94.5	51.8	0–266
	Cerec†	177.1	84.7	44–332	160.3	97.0	0–384
	Mirage‡	88.2	2.4	0–306	144.0	109.5	38–505
	Empress§	121.8	97.5	0–626	139.7	81.4	21–326
Occlusal area	Gold	29.9	37.9	0–153	57.1	40.6	0–193
	Cerec†	131.4	92.3	0–355	123.4	87.0	0–369
	Mirage‡	51.6	53.6	0–261	48.5	53.9	0–221
	Empress§	65.7	70.0	0–427	93.8	69.4	0–413

From Molin and Karlsson [28••]; with permission.
†Siemens Dental Corp., Bensheim, FRG.
‡Myron, Kansas City, KS.
§Ivoclar, Amherst, NY.

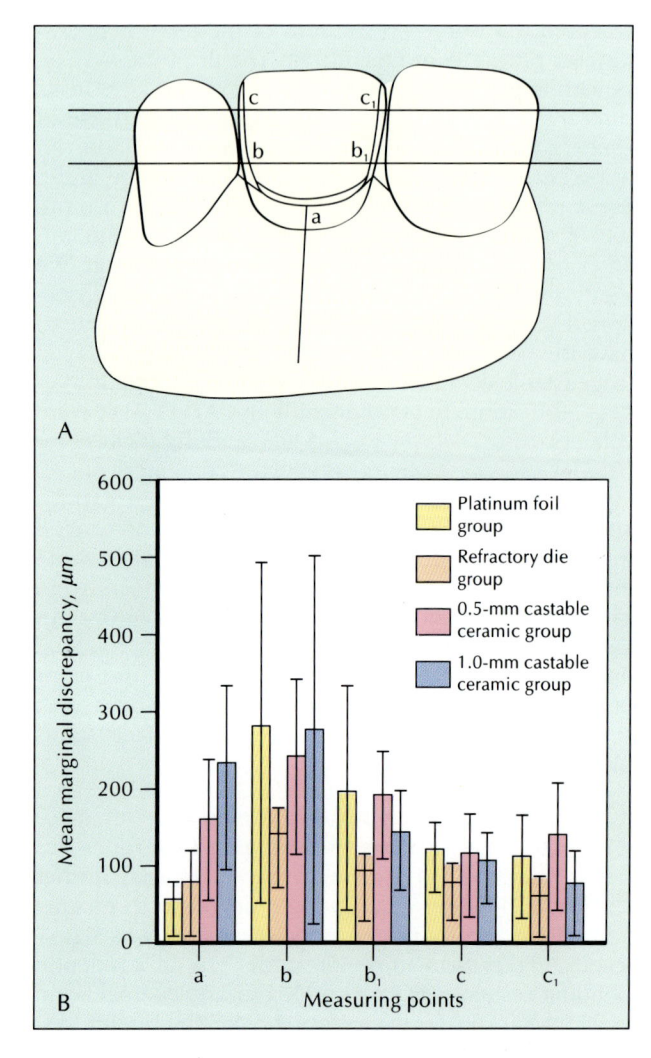

Fig. 2. A, Locations of sectioning. Point *a* indicates midlabial margin. Points *b* and *b₁* define the gingival horizontal section. Points *c* and *c₁* define the incisal horizontal section. **B,** Fit of the veneers at the five locations. *T bars* indicate SD. (*From* Sim and Ibbetson [31]; with permission.)

appears that it is still best to do what we can to keep the preparation in enamel as much as possible. Regarding the technical fabrication of the veneers themselves, Sheets and Taniguchi [35] described a new multidie technique with removable refractory dies in a master stone cast that allowed different types of restorations in a complex treatment plan to be fabricated at the same time.

As for the clinical prognosis of veneers, in an excellent and important study, Dunne and Millar [36••] evaluated 315 porcelain veneers over a 5-year period. Although there were many variables—some veneers were placed in different clinics and by different operators (including students); some were made by different techniques (foil refractory dies); some were bonded with and without rubber dam—after 5 years, of the 315 that were followed up, 262 (83%) remained problem-free. It appears that despite the many clinical variables, porcelain veneers are an effective and reliable treatment modality.

Crowns

The porcelain-fused-to-metal (PFM) crown has long been the full crown standard and is still regarded by some as the best choice for full-coverage posterior restorations [37••]. Improving the technical aspects of the metal system is still a goal [38,39] as is improving the esthetics of PFM crowns by eliminating the gold collar and using a butt porcelain shoulder [40]. Still, there remains the problem of the lack of translucency of a metal-opaquer-porcelain system that tends to give a less than natural look to PFM crowns [41•] and has lead to the development of several all-porcelain alternatives.

Aside from the obvious importance of esthetics, several factors are essential to the success of anterior and posterior all-ceramic crowns: porcelain strength, marginal design and integrity, luting technique, and modulus of elasticity of the understructure, to name a few.

Vita In-Ceram (Vita Zahnfabrik) is generally acknowledged to be the strongest porcelain available [37••,41•, 42]. It is a closely packed, sintered alumina framework [43] infiltrated in a second step with molten glass. Although it is so dense that it cannot be traditionally etched and bonded to the tooth structure, its natural fracture resistance has been clinically demonstrated in a 35-month study of 61 anterior and posterior crowns, none of which failed, although they had been luted with traditional zinc phosphate cement [42]. Another study of a magnesia core crown covered with different body porcelains reported that the magnesia core crown was stronger than a comparable Hi-Ceram (Vita Zahnfabrik) aluminous core crown and significantly stronger than a Renaissance crown (Williams Gold, Buffalo, NY) (porcelain fired over a swaged heat-treated foil) [44]. Pressure-molded Empress crowns obtained the proper shades from two techniques: surface staining and a veneer technique. Lüthy *et al.* [45] found that there was no significant difference in flexure strength using either technique, and using the strength of Empress, its castability, esthetics, and ability to be etched and bonded to tooth, Freedman [46] described using it for a cast post and core under ceramic crowns. Studying the effect of different luting media (*ie*, zinc phosphate, glass ionomer, and resin cements) on etched but unsilanated and unbonded Hi-Ceram and Dicor castable ceramic crowns, McCormack *et al.* [47] found that the type of cement had no significant effect on the compressive strength of the crowns. When Dicor was etched, silanated, and bonded to the tooth in a similar study, however, the resin-bonded crowns were significantly stronger than the cemented crowns (Table 2), even counteracting the potentially weakening effect of different finish line designs [48•]. Further complicating the sophisticated topic of crown strength, Scherrer and Rijk

[49] found that even the modulus of elasticity of the supporting structure may have a significant effect on the fracture resistance of all-ceramic crowns.

Table 2. Effect of cement on strength of 15 ceramic crowns using finish line with shoulder and 0.3 mm of axiogingival rounding*

Cement type†	Breaking strength, kg ± SD
Visible light–activated resin	142.73 ± 21.68
Glass-ionomer	104.80 ± 21.28‡
Zinc phosphate	98.33 ± 20.61‡

*From Bernal et al. [48•]; with permission.
†Listed in decreasing order of restoration strength.
‡Values are not significantly different at the 95% confidence level (Newman-Keul's test).

As with almost any other dental restoration, the fit of the full porcelain crown is important to its long-range clinical success. Measuring porcelain-fused-to-Dicor accuracy, using chamfer, a 45° bevel, and 90° shoulder marginal designs, Hoard et al. [50] found no significant difference in marginal adaptation. Despite the findings, however, they believed the 45° bevel should be used with caution. Finally, studying the marginal accuracy of a full platinum foil, a modified platinum foil, and a refractory die fabrication of a magnesia-core porcelain crown, Mora et al. [51•] found a significant difference between the techniques: a mean marginal opening of 57.2 ± 26.3 µm for the conventional platinum foil, 32.8 ± 13.4 µm for the modified foil, and 22.1 ± 20.4 µm for the refractory technique.

Fixed partial dentures

The extensive preparation required and the lack of esthetic "aliveness" in PFM fixed partial dentures (FPDs) has resulted in several different approaches to replacing missing teeth. Rochette and Maryland metal wing bridges were introduced for this purpose, but have not proved to be as durable as hoped [52]; in addition, the metal caused esthetic problems. As bonding procedures and porcelain strength have significantly improved, metal-free full- and partial-coverage FPDs of different designs have been developed.

Using a labial porcelain veneer abutment preparation, Dennisen et al. [53] reported a 75% success rate after 5 years for 12 all-porcelain FPDs of unspecified porcelain material. In-Ceram has been the porcelain used most for FPDs because of its high fracture strength. Using full shoulder preparations and conventional zinc phosphate cement, Pröbster [42] found 13 of 15 In-Ceram FPDs were still in service after 35 months, attesting to the potential for these restorations. Using a more conservative lingual preparation, Kern et al. [54] tested the in vitro resistance to fracture of In-Ceram FPDs, bonded (using a special silica- and silane-coated Rocatec system [ESPE, Seefeld, FRG] with Panavia-TC [J. Morita, Tustin, CA] adhesive resin) to extracted teeth with and without an artificial periodontal ligament [54]. All of the fractures occurred at the connector between the pontic and the wings, and the presence of the artificial periodontal ligament did not reduce the fracture strength of the bridges. In another study, they found that the addition of a proximal box to the lingual preparation and veneering the pontic with Vitadur N porcelain circumferentially instead of just labially significantly improved the fracture strength of the In-Ceram FPDs [55] (Fig. 3). Thermocycling and storing the FPDs for 150 days in artificial saliva significantly reduced the fracture strength, although, in a clinically significant finding, the measured fracture strengths remained within range of the normal physiologic forces seen in the anterior region. Finally, using porcelain as a pontic veneering material, Serio [56] described a conservative FPD bonded composite bridge design (the Encore Bridge; Da Vinci Laboratory, Woodland Hills, CA), that, because of its flexibility in relation to rigid porcelain, may distribute a more favorable load transfer to bone and the abutment teeth.

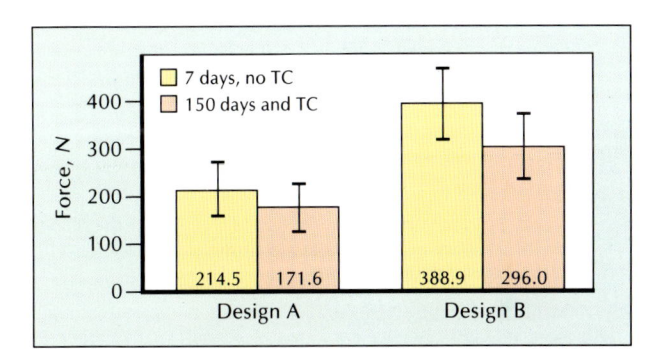

Fig. 3. Forces required to fracture resin-bonded In-Ceram (Vident, Baldwin Park, CA) ceramic fixed partial dentures. TC—thermal cycling. T bars indicate SD. (From Kern et al. [55]; with permission.)

Conclusions

Porcelain has been an important material in restorative dentistry for many years because of its wearability and esthetic qualities, but until recently, its use, unsupported by a rigid metal framework, was limited to relatively weak, poorly fitting porcelain jacket crowns cemented on extensively prepared anterior teeth. Two developments have changed how we think about all-porcelain restorations, however, and have expanded the use of metal-free ceramics to all areas of the mouth. First, the development of very effective resin bonding techniques and materials has allowed us to become more conservative in tooth preparation and more adventurous in how and where we use porcelain in the mouth. Second, the development of better fitting and much stronger porcelains has hinted at a future of highly esthetic ceramic restorations that may allow us to be more creative as cosmetic dentists and to better fulfill the needs and desires of our patients.

References and recommended reading

Papers of particular interest, published within the annual period of review, have been highlighted as:
- Of special interest
- • Of outstanding interest

1. Widström E, Haugejorden O, Sundberg H, Birn H: **Nordic dentists' opinions on the safety of amalgam and other dental restorative materials.** *Scand J Dent Res* 1993, 101:238–242.

2. Bagambisa F, Kappert H, Schilli W: **Interfacial reactions of odontoblasts to dental and implant materials.** *J Oral Maxillofac Surg* 1994, 52:52–56.

3. Baker P, Clark A: **Compositional influence on the strength of dental porcelain.** *Int J Prosthodont* 1993, 6:291–297.

4. Kon M, Kuwayama N: **Effect of adding diamond particles on the fracture toughness of apatite ceramics.** *Dent Mater J* 1993, 12:12–17.

5. Denry I, Rosenstiel J, Holloway J, Niemiec M: **Enhanced chemical strengthening of feldspathic dental porcelain.** *J Dent Res* 1993, 72:1429–1433.

6. Denry I, Rosenstiel J: **Flexural strength and fracture toughness of Dicor glass-ceramic after embedment modification.** *J Dent Res* 1993, 72:572–576.

7. Hojjatie B, Anusavice K: **Effects of initial temperature and tempering medium on thermal tempering of dental porcelains.** *J Dent Res* 1993, 72:556–571.

8. Akkas S: **Prediction of the service life of dental porcelains by the measurements of post-indentation slow crack growth.** *Dent Mater J* 1993, 12:45–53.

9. Mante F, Brantley W, Dhuru V, Ziebert G: **Fracture toughness of high alumina core dental ceramics: the effect of water and artificial saliva.** *Int J Prosthodont* 1993, 6:546–552.

10. Thompson J, Anusavice K: **Effect of surface etching on the flexure strength and fracture toughness of Dicor disks containing controlled flaws.** *J Dent Res* 1994, 73:505–510.

11. Yen T, Blackman R, Baez R: **Effect of acid etching on the**
• **flexural strength of a feldspathic porcelain and a castable glass ceramic.** *J Prosthet Dent* 1993, 70:224–233.
A good study of a very basic procedure in dental bonding interspersed with a detailed discussion of feldspathic porcelain and castable glass ceramic chemistry.

12. Hahn R, Löst C: **Microstructure and strength analysis of ultrasonically shaped ceramics.** *Schweiz Monatsschr Zahnmed* 1993, 103:844–850.

13. Russell D, Meiers J: **Shear bond strength of resin compos-**
•• **ite to Dicor treated with 4 META.** *Int J Prosthodont* 1994, 7:7–12.
A clinically important study of different surface treatments and chemical bonding agents, stressing the importance of micromechanical (especially etching) retention for a significantly stronger bond.

14. Suliman A, Swift E, Perdigao J: **Effects of surface treatment**
•• **and bonding agents on bond strength of composite resin to porcelain.** *J Prosthet Dent* 1993, 70:118–120.
A very interesting study of several porcelain repair surface treatments and bonding agents. It stresses the importance of surface roughening (the most effective being diamond bur and hydrofluoric acid in combination) and silanation for the most effective bonding.

15. Ekfeldt A, Fransson B, Söderlund B, Øilo G: **Wear resistance of some prosthodontic materials in vivo.** *Acta Odontol Scand* 1993, 51:99–107.

16. Hulterström A, Bergman M: **Polishing systems for dental ceramics.** *Acta Odontol Scand* 1993, 51:229–234.

17. Scurria M, Powers J: **Surface roughness of two polished ceramic materials.** *J Prosthet Dent* 1994, 71:174–177.

18. Monsénégo G, Burdairon G, Clerjaud B: **Fluorescence of dental porcelain.** *J Prosthet Dent* 1993, 69:106–113.

19. Donovan T, Chee W: **Conservative indirect restorations for posterior teeth.** *Dent Clin North Am* 1993, 37:433–443.

20. Burke F, Qualtrough A: **Aesthetic inlays: composite or ceramic?** *Br Dent J* 1993, 176:53–60.

21. Blair K, Koeppen R, Schwartz R, Davis R: **Microleakage associated with resin composite-cemented, cast glass ceramic restoration.** *Int J Prosthodont* 1993, 6:579–584.

22. Peters M, De Vree J, Brekelmans W: **Distributed crack analysis of ceramic inlays.** *J Dent Res* 1993, 72:1537–1542.

23. Krejci I, Lutz F, Reimer M, Heinzmann J: **Wear of ceramic inlays, their enamel antagonists, and luting cements.** *J Prosthet Dent* 1993, 69:425–430.

24. O'Neal S, Miracle R, Leinfelder K: **Evaluating interfacial gaps**
•• **for esthetic inlays.** *J Am Dent Assoc* 1993, 124:48–54.
An important study of the fit of two resin and two ceramic inlay systems and the wear of the bonding material. In essence, the better the fit, the less the cement wear gap.

25. Rekow E: **High-technology innovations—and imitations—for**
• **restorative dentistry.** *Dent Clin North Am* 1993, 37:513–524.
Contains a brief but detailed description of the state of CAD-CAM technology.

26. Shearer A, Heymann H, Wilson N: **Two ceramic materials compared for the production of CEREC inlays.** *J Dent* 1993, 21:302–304.

27. Nathanson D, Riis D, Cataldo G, Ashayeri N: **CAD-CAM ce-**
• **ramic inlays and onlays: using an indirect technique.** *J Am Dent Assoc* 1994, 125:421–427.
A detailed description of the CAD-CAM process and technique from the standpoint of its use as a "mini-lab" for an indirect porcelain inlay technique.

28. Molin M, Karlsson S: **The fit of gold inlays and three ceramic**
•• **inlay systems.** *Acta Odontol Scand* 1993, 51:201–206.
A well-designed study comparing the inlay marginal fit of gold and Cerec, Mirage, and Empress ceramics both on a die and on the tooth. As expected, the gold inlay fit best, and Cerec showed the largest marginal discrepancies. Of particular interest were the large standard deviations, particularly for the ceramic systems, indicating a microscopically rough surface.

29. Stenberg R, Matsson L: **Clinical evaluation of glass ceramic inlays (Dicor).** *Acta Odontol Scand* 1993, 51:91–97.

30. McIntyre F, Bochiechio R, Johnson R: **Marginal gap width of a new refractory porcelain system.** *J Prosthet Dent* 1993, 69:564–567.

31. Sim C, Ibbetson R: **Comparison of fit of porcelain veneers fabricated using different techniques.** *Int J Prosthodont* 1993, 6:36–42.

32. Liu P, Isenberg B, Leinfelder K: **Evaluating CAD-CAM generated ceramic veneers.** *J Am Dent Assoc* 1993, 124:59–63.

33. Barnes D, Gingell J, Blank L: **One-year clinical evaluation of porcelain veneers.** *Esthet Dent Update* 1993, 4:111–115.

34. Barkmeier W, Menis D, Barnes D: **Bond strength of a veneering porcelain using newer generation adhesive systems.** *Pract Periodontics Aesthet Dent* 1993, 5:50–55.

35. Sheets C, Taniguchi T: **A multidie technique for the fabrication of porcelain laminate veneers.** *J Prosthet Dent* 1993, 70:291–295.

36. Dunne S, Millar B: **A longitudinal study of the clinical performance of porcelain veneers.** *Br Dent J* 1993, **175**:317–321.

•• An excellent large-sample, long-range study of the effects of various factors on the success and failure rates of 315 porcelain veneers placed in two teaching hospitals. With differences in operators, fabrication techniques, use of rubber dam, and reason for placement, to name a few, the success rate was 83%.

37. Anusavice K: **Recent developments in restorative dental ceramics.** *J Am Dent Assoc* 1993, **124**:72–84.

•• An excellent review and evaluation of the latest developments in porcelain technology with an extensive table of the relative strengths of 13 different porcelains.

38. Papazoglou E, Brantley W, Carr A, Johnston W: **Porcelain adherence to high-palladium alloys.** *J Prosthet Dent* 1993, **70**:386–394.

39. Karlsson S: **The fit of Procera titanium crowns.** *Acta Odontol Scand* 1993, **51**:129–134.

40. Boyle J, Naylor W, Blackman R: **Marginal accuracy of metal ceramic restorations with porcelain facial margins.** *J Prosthet Dent* 1993, **69**:19–27.

41. Christensen G: **Ceramic vs porcelain-fused-to-metal crowns: give your patients a choice.** *J Am Dent Assoc* 1994, **125**:311–314.

• A concise summary of the range of porcelain products available.

42. Pröbster L: **Survival rate of In-Ceram restorations.** *Int J Prosthodont* 1993, **6**:259–263.

43. Andersson M, Odén A: **A new all-ceramic crown.** *Acta Odontol Scand* 1993, **51**:59–64.

44. Liu C, O'Brien W: **Strength of magnesia-core crown with different body porcelains.** *Int J Prosthodont* 1993, **6**:60–64.

45. Lüthy H, Dong J, Wohlwend A, Schärer P: **Effects of veneering and glazing on the strength of heat-pressed ceramics.** *Schweiz Monatsschr Zahnmed* 1993, **103**:1257–1260.

46. Freedman G: **Castable ceramic post/cores and crowns.** *Dent Econ* 1993, **83**:90–91.

47. McCormick J, Rowland W, Schillingburg H, Duncanson M: **Effect of luting media on the compressive strengths of two types of all-ceramic crown.** *Quintessence Int* 1993, **24**:405–408.

48. Bernal G, Jones R, Brown D, Munoz C, Goodacre C: **The effect of finish line form and luting agent on the breaking strength of Dicor crowns.** *Int J Prosthodont* 1993, **6**:286–290.

• A well-designed study of clinical relevance showing the effects of bonding versus cementing ceramics.

49. Scherrer S, Rijk W: **The fracture resistance of all-ceramic crowns on supporting structures with different elastic moduli.** *Int J Prosthodont* 1993, **6**:462–467.

50. Hoard R, Chiang P, Hewlett E, Caputo A: **Marginal discrepancy as related to marginal design in porcelain-fused-to-Dicor restorations.** *Oral Health* 1993, March:15–18.

51. Mora G, O'Brien W, Lazar E: **Marginal fit of all-ceramic core crowns made with platinum foil and refractory die methods.** *Esthet Dent Update* 1993, **4**:138–142.

• A summary of the marginal fit of various new ceramic systems as well as a discussion of how platinum foil versus refractory die fabrication of ceramic crowns can significantly affect marginal fit.

52. Berekally T, Smales R: **A retrospective clinical evaluation of resin-bonded bridges inserted at the Adelaide Dental Hospital.** *Aust Dent J* 1993, **38**:85–96.

53. Denissen H, Wijnhoff G, Veldhuis A, Kalk W: **Five-year study of all-porcelain veneer fixed partial dentures.** *J Prosthet Dent* 1993, **69**:464–468.

54. Kern M, Douglas W, Fechtig T, Strub J, DeLong R: **Fracture strength of all-porcelain, resin-bonded bridges after testing in an artificial oral environment.** *J Dent* 1993, **21**:117–121.

55. Kern M, Fechtig T, Strub J: **Influence of water storage and thermal cycling on the fracture strength of all-porcelain, resin-bonded fixed partial dentures.** *J Prosthet Dent* 1994, **71**:251–256.

56. Serio A: **Composite bridges: pros and cons.** *Esthet Dent Update* 1993, **6**:150–151.

David M. Schneider, DMD, MScD, 990 Paradise Road, Swampscott, MA 01907, USA.

Index to subjects

Abrams roll technique, in ridge augmentation, 19
Acid etching
  for adhesion, 69–71
  of porcelain, 58, 63
    for repair, 89
Adhesion systems, 69–74
  for dentin, 70–72
  for enamel, 69–70
  etching in, 69–71
  for gap-free restorations, 71
  history of, 69–70
  hybrid layer formation in, 71–72
  for porcelain veneers see under Porcelain veneers
  wet bonding in, 72
Advertising, 104–105
Aging
  dentition changes with, restoration of, 41–44
  marketing and, 102–103
All-Bond system, for restoration repair, 89–90
Amalgambond, for restoration repair, 89
Anesthesia, for porcelain veneers, 46
Antibiotics, in periodontal disease, 44
Argon laser, clinical applications of, 94
Association, in esthetic dentistry, 25, 27

Balance, in esthetic dentistry, 29
Banking, tooth, porcelain onlays for, 1–2
Barrier membranes, for gingival recession, 19
Beauty, in esthetic dentistry, 24–27
Benzalkonium chloride, in etching gels, 70
Bleaching, in disharmony treatment, 33
Bonding
  to dentin, 62–63, 70–72
  wet, 72
  see also Adhesion systems

Camfer's line, as reference, in impression system, 82
Carbon dioxide laser, clinical applications of, 93
Cementation
  of composite restorations, 54–55
  of porcelain veneers, 64–65
Cements, for porcelain veneers, 49
Ceramic restorations
  repair of, 89–91
  see also Porcelain
Cerec system, in ceramic restoration design and manufacture, 108
Clearfil Porcelain Bond, for restoration repair, 89–90
Color
  darkening of, in aging dentition, 41–42
  management of
    bleaching in, 33
    porcelain veneer matching in, 33–34, 46–47, 63–64, 108
    science of, 36–37
    selection technique in, 37–39
    shade-matching environment in, 37
    in tetracycline-stained teeth, 39
    veneer-crown matching in, 34–35
Colorlogic porcelain veneer material, 108–109
Common preparation, for porcelain veneers, 45–46
Composite resins
  for onlays, 6
  for porcelain veneers, 60–61, 108
Composite restorations
  indirect, 51–56
  advantages of, 51–52
  cementation of, 54–55
  indications for, 52
  materials for, 52
  preparation of, 53–54
  laser curing of, 97–98
  repair of, 90
Computers
  in ceramic restoration design and manufacture, 108–109
  in consultation visit, 76–77
  in diagnosis, 12, 16, 76
  in impression system, 85
  in record maintenance, 75–76
  in treatment, 77–78
  in treatment planning, 76
Concept composite resins, 52
Connective tissue autograft
  for gingival recession, 18–19
  for ridge augmentation, 19
Conservation, of tooth, porcelain onlays for, 1
Content, in esthetic dentistry, 27
Crowns
  matching of, with porcelain veneers, 34–35
  porcelain, 110–111
Cultural biases, in esthetics, 24–25

Dental view, in esthetic diagnosis, 11–12
Dentin
  bonding systems for, 62–63, 70–72
  cutting of, lasers in, 94
  sclerosis of, in aging, 42
Dentofacial references, in impression system, 80–81
Dentofacial view, in esthetic diagnosis, 10–12
Dentures, partial fixed, porcelain in, 111
Diagnosis, esthetic see Esthetics, diagnosis in
Dicor
  for crowns, 110–111
  for inlays and onlays, 108
Disharmony, treatment of, 33–35
Disinfection, for adhesion systems, 70
Distortion, in esthetic dentistry, 25
Dominance, in esthetic dentistry, 29
Duceram LFC system, for onlays, 6

Economy, in esthetic dentistry, 29
Elderly persons
  dentition changes in, restoration techniques for, 41–44
  marketing directed to, 102–103
Empress system
  for crowns, 110
  for onlays, 4–6, 108
Enamel
  cutting of, lasers in, 94
  etching of, for adhesion, 69–70
Erbium laser, clinical applications of, 94
Esthetics
  diagnosis in, 9–17
    common language in, 10–12
    therapeutic mind set in, 9–10
    three-step analysis in, 12, 16
    wax-up in, 16
  periodontal therapy in, 18–23
  visual arts and, 24–32
    beauty, 24–27
    clinical applications of, 30–32
    content, 27

114

principles of organization, 27–29
subject, 27
unity, 27
Etching
for adhesion, 69–71
of porcelain, 58, 63
for repair, 89

Face
alterations of, with aging, 42–43
impression of, 82
Facebow transfer technique, 83
Facial view, in esthetic diagnosis, 10
Forming, visual, in esthetic dentistry, 27–28
Fractures, of restorations, repair of, 89–91
Free gingival autograft, for gingival recession, 18–19

Gels, for etching, 70
Gingiva
laser surgery on, 94–98
recession of, grafts for, 18–19, 42
symmetry of, in esthetic diagnosis, 11
Grafts
for gingival recession, 18–19, 42
onlay, in ridge augmentation, 19

Harmony, in esthetic dentistry, 28–29, 33–35
Hemostasis, lasers in, 94
Holmium laser, clinical applications of, 94
Hybrid layer, in adhesion systems, 71–72
Hydrofluoric acid
in composite etching, 90
in porcelain etching, 89

Impression system, 80–88
computer imaging in, 85
contraindications for, 86
dentofacial references in, 80–81
functional references in, 81
indications for, 85–86
laboratory procedures in, 83–84
lip reproduction in, 81–82, 85–87
in orthognathic surgical planning, 86–87
photographs in, 85
putty core index in, 85
restorative treatment procedures after, 82–85
three-dimensional fabrication references in, 81
two-dimensional linear references in, 81
for veneers, 47
In-Ceram
for crowns, 110
for fixed partial dentures, 111
Inlays and onlays, 1–8
application of, 2
ceramic selection for, 4–6
composite resins for, 6
design of, 2–4
fit of, 2
occlusion fine-tuning with, 6–7
predictability of, 1
preparations for, 108–109
sequencing of, 7
in tooth conservation, 1
in tooth strengthening, 1–2
Interpupillary line, as reference, in impression system, 82
Intuition, in esthetic dentistry, 25

Kalco System, for lip reproduction, 81–82

Lasers, 92–99
clinical applications of
advantages of, 92
case study of, 94–98
vs. laser type, 93–94
historical review of, 92–93
principles of, 92
Light, for color matching, 37
Lips
contour alterations of, with aging, 43
as references, in impression system, 80–81
reproduction of, in impression system, 81–82, 85–87
Luting agents
in color correction, 33–34
composite resin, for porcelain veneers, 60, 62
for crowns, 110

Marketing, 100–106
advertising in, 104–105
demographic studies for, 102–103
external, 101
internal, 100–101
Metal restorations, repair of, 90
Microleakage, prevention of, total etch technique in, 71
Moist bonding systems, 72

Neodymium:yttrium-aluminum-garnet laser, clinical applications of, 93–94

Occlusion
alterations of, with aging, 43
fine-tuning of, with porcelain onlays, 6–7
Onlay grafting, in ridge augmentation, 19
Onlays see Inlays and onlays
Optec HSP, for onlays, 4
Optibond dentin bonding agent, 62
Oral hygiene, surface wear from, 43
Ordering, visual, in esthetic dentistry, 27–28
Orthognathic surgical planning, impression system for, 86–87

Papilla, interdental, preservation of, 19–21
Parallel ruler, in facebow alignment, 83
Partial dentures, fixed, porcelain in, 111
Pedicle graft
laterally positioned, for gingival recession, 18–19
for ridge augmentation, 19
Periodontics, 18–23
antibiotic cords in, 44
interdental papilla preservation in, 19–21
lasers in, 94–98
ridge augmentation in, 19
root coverage in, 18–19
Permagen dentin bonding agent, 62
Phonetics, as reference, in impression system, 82
Phosphoric acid, for etching, 70–71
Photographs, in restoration, 85
Piezoelectric scalers, 43–44
Plastic surgery, periodontal, 18–23
Polishing, of porcelain, 108
Porcelain, 107–113
composite resin bonding to, 108
for crowns, 110–111
esthetic advantages of, 108
in fixed partial dentures, 111
for inlays and onlays see Porcelain inlays and onlays
polishing of, 108
repair of, 89–91
research on, 107–108
for veneers see Porcelain veneers
Porcelain inlays and onlays, 1–8

application of, 2
ceramic selection for, 4–6
composite resins for, 6
design of, 2–4
fit of, 2
occlusion fine-tuning with, 6–7
predictability of, 1
preparations for, 108
sequencing of, 7
in tooth conservation, 1
in tooth strengthening, 1–2
Porcelain veneers
adhesion systems for, 49, 57–68, 108
cementation of, 64–65
components of, 58–63
durability of, 63
future of, 65–66
history of, 57
shading in, 63–64
temporization in, 63
durability of, 110
etching of, 58, 63
fitting of, 109
matching of, 33–34
with crowns, 34–35
materials for, 109–110
preparation of
anesthesia for, 46
common, 45–46
impression in, 47
placement in, 47–49
shade selection in, 46–47
slice, 46
temporization in, 47, 63
tooth reduction in, 46
window, 46
pretreatment considerations with, 45
for tetracycline staining, 39, 94–98
Pouch procedures, in ridge augmentation, 19
Primers, for dentin bonding, 62–63
Pulp, etching effects on, 71
Putty core index, 85

Repair, of restorations, 89–91
Resins
composite *see* Composite resins; Composite restorations
luting *see* Luting agents
Restorations
repair of, 89–91
see also Composite restorations

Ridge augmentation, 19
Roll technique, in ridge augmentation, 19
Roots
coverage of, 18–19
sensitivity of, in elderly persons, 42

Scalers, piezoelectric, 43–44
ScotchBond dentin bonding agents, 62–65
Semigels, for etching, 70
Silane coupling, of porcelain veneers, 58
Slice preparation, for porcelain veneers, 46
Smile
aging effects on, 41–42
treatment of, 42–44
esthetics of *see* Esthetics
impression of, 82, 85–86
Sodium gels, neutral, for sensitivity, 44
Spinell material, for onlays, 6
Staining
from food and beverages, 42
tetracycline
color management of, 39
porcelain veneers for, 94–98
Strengthening, of tooth, porcelain onlays for, 1–2
Subject, in esthetic dentistry, 27
Surface texture, alterations of, with aging, 43

Technology, 75–79
in consultation visit, 76–77
in diagnosis, 76
for new patient visit, 75–76
in treatment, 77–78
in treatment planning, 76
see also Computers
Temporization, in porcelain veneer placement, 47, 63
Temporomandibular joint surgery, lasers in, 94
Tenure dentin bonding agent, 62
Tetracycline-stained teeth
color management of, 39
porcelain veneers for, 94–98
Total etch procedures, 70–71

Unity, in esthetic dentistry, 27

Variety, in esthetic dentistry, 25, 28–29
Veneers, porcelain *see* Porcelain veneers
Video, in high-tech office, 76–77
Visual arts, in esthetic dentistry *see under* Esthetics

Wet bonding systems, 72
Whitening, in disharmony treatment, 33
Window preparation, for porcelain veneers, 46